CPC CODING QUICK GUIDE

Essential Exam Review

APARAJITA SUDARSHAN

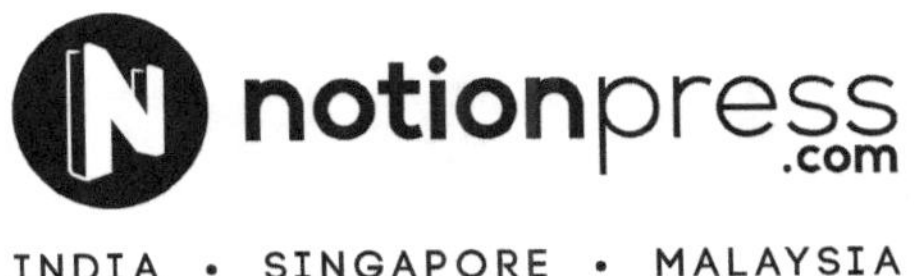

notionpress.com

INDIA • SINGAPORE • MALAYSIA

ISBN
Hardcase 979-8-89556-634-3
Paperback 979-8-89544-536-5

Contents

Contents

Acknowledgement

This book marks a significant milestone in my journey, and I hope it serves as a valuable contribution to all the budding medical coders out there. I wish each of you the very best in your endeavours.

First and foremost, I want to thank God for giving me the strength to see this project through to completion. Without his guidance, this achievement would not have been possible.

I am deeply grateful to my parents, Mr. Anup K. De and Mrs. Swagata De, who have walked this journey with me. They raised me both as a son and a daughter, with a perfect balance of gentleness and firmness. Their unwavering support, tough love, and refusal to let me give up, even when life and circumstances seemed overwhelming, have been invaluable. Thank you for always believing in me and for nurturing the resilience that has carried me through.

To my children, Ved and Ira, your love and light keep me going every day. You inspire me to be the best version of myself.

Lastly, my deepest thanks go to my husband, Sudarshan Ravindran. You have helped me dream bigger and work harder every single day. You push me beyond my limits, always surprising me with new challenges, knowing full well that, together, we can overcome anything. Your belief in me has been my greatest strength.

I dedicate this book to you, my partner, Sudarshan, for your endless support, love, and encouragement. This achievement is as much yours as it is mine.

Aparajita Sudarshan

DISCLAIMER:

The questions featured at the end of each chapter are compiled from a variety of sources, including established study manuals. The content has been carefully selected and restructured to enhance clarity and accessibility. While the questions are based on industry-standard guidelines, the organization and presentation are the result of my own editorial efforts. This work is intended to provide a practical and user-friendly resource for readers, and is not meant to claim originality of the content sourced from other publications.

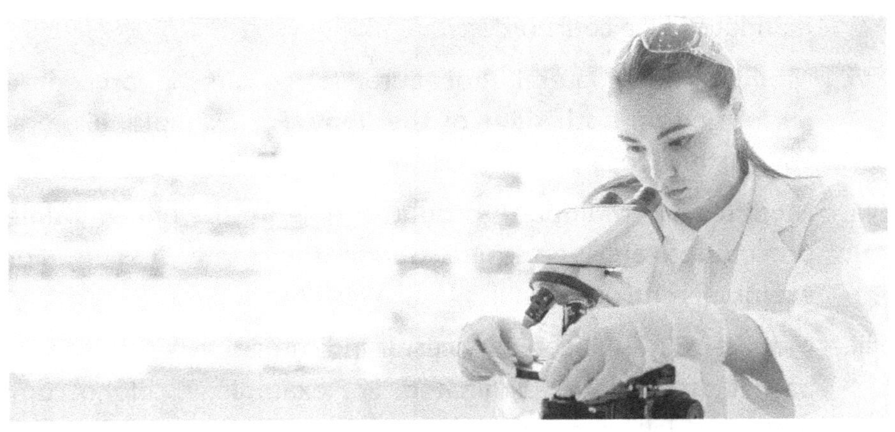

i.   **Modifier 22**: Increased Procedural Services. It indicates that the work required to perform a service is substantially **greater than typically required**. **For example,** a surgeon encounters unexpected extensive adhesions during a laparotomy.

ii. **Modifier 24:** Unrelated Evaluation and Management Service by the **Same Physician During a Postoperative Period.** It is used for an E/M service unrelated to the original procedure. **For example,** a patient returns with a cold 10 days after surgery.

iii. **Modifier 25:** Significant, Separately Identifiable E/M Service by the **Same Physician on the Same Day of the Procedure or Other Service.** It indicates a separate E/M service on the same day as another procedure. **For example,** a patient is seen for hypertension and also receives a vaccine.

iv. **Modifier 26:** It is used for professional component. It is used when only the **professional component** of a service is performed. **For example,** a radiologist interprets an X-ray but does not provide the technical component.

v. **Modifier 32: Mandated Services.** It is used when services are required by a third party. For example, a physical exam mandated by a court order.

vi. **Modifier 50:** Bilateral Procedure. It indicates a procedure performed on **both sides of the body.** For example, bilateral knee arthroscopy.

vii. **Modifier 51:** Multiple Procedures. It is used when **multiple procedures** are performed during the same session. **For example,** removal of multiple skin lesions.

viii. **Modifier 52:** Reduced Services. It indicates that a service was partially reduced or eliminated. **For example,** a colonoscopy that is partially completed due to patient intolerance.

ix. **Modifier 53:** Discontinued Procedure. It indicates that a procedure was discontinued. **For example, surgery halted** due to patient's cardiac arrest.

x. **Modifier 54:** Surgical Care Only. It is used when only the surgical care is provided. **For example,** a surgeon performs surgery, but another physician handles pre- and post-operative care.

xi. **Modifier 55:** Postoperative Management Only. It is used when postoperative care is provided by a different physician than the surgeon. **For example,** follow-up care by a family physician after surgery.

xii. **Modifier 56:** Preoperative Management Only. It is used when preoperative care is provided by a different physician than the surgeon. **For example,** preoperative evaluation by an internist.

xiii. **Modifier 57:** Decision for Surgery. It indicates an E/M service that resulted in the initial decision to perform surgery. **For example,** an initial consultation leads to immediate surgery.

xiv. **Modifier 58:** Staged or related procedure or service by the same physician during the postoperative period. It indicates a staged or related procedure during the postoperative period. **For example,** a planned second stage of surgery.

xv. **Modifier 59:** Distinct Procedural Service. It indicates services that are not normally reported together but are appropriate under the circumstances. **For example**, a patient has two separate skin lesions removed.

xvi. **Modifier 62:** Two Surgeons. It indicates a procedure performed by **two surgeons. For example,** two surgeons performing a complex cardiovascular surgery.

xvii. **Modifier 76:** Repeat Procedure by Same Physician. It indicates **a repeat procedure by the same physician. For example,** a follow-up angiogram performed the same day due to complications.

xviii. **Modifier 77:** Repeat Procedure by Another Physician. It indicates a **repeat procedure** by a different physician. **For example,** another surgeon performs a follow-up endoscopy due to complications.

xix. **Modifier 78:** Unplanned Return to the Operating/Procedure Room by the Same Physician Following Initial Procedure for a Related Procedure During the Postoperative Period. **For example,** emergency surgery for postoperative bleeding.

xx. **Modifier 79**: Unrelated Procedure or Service by the Same Physician During the Postoperative Period. For example, a new, unrelated surgery during the postoperative period of a previous surgery.

xxi. **Modifier 80:** Assistant Surgeon. It is used when an **assistant surgeon is required. For example,** a secondary surgeon assists in a complex operation.

xxii. **Modifier 90:** Reference (Outside) Laboratory. It indicates that laboratory procedures were performed by an outside lab. For example, blood tests sent to an external lab for analysis.

xxiii. **Modifier 91:** Repeat Clinical Diagnostic Laboratory Test. **For example,** multiple blood glucose tests in one day to monitor levels.

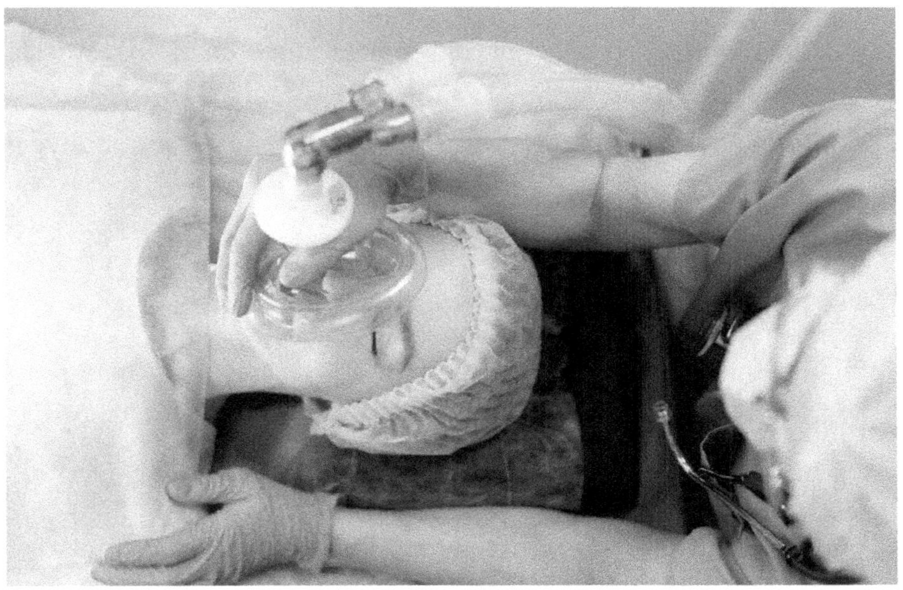

Anaesthesia Codes Range: 00100-01999: Used to report anaesthesia services.

Anaesthesia Type:

i.   **General Anaesthesia**: Complete unconsciousness.

ii. **Regional Anaesthesia**: Numbs a large part of the body.

iii. **Monitored Anaesthesia Care (MAC)**: Conscious sedation with a focus on patient safety and comfort.

iv. **Local Anaesthesia**: Numbs a small area.

Reporting Anaesthesia Time:

- **Start to End**: Time is reported from when the anaesthesiologist begins preparing the patient to when the patient is no longer under the provider's care.
- **Minutes**: Anaesthesia time is typically documented in minutes.

Base Units and Time Units:

- **Base Units**: Reflect the complexity of the service.
- **Time Units**: Typically one unit per 15 minutes of anaesthesia time.
- **Total Anaesthesia Units**: Base units + time units + any modifying units.

Example To Calculate Total Anaesthesia Time

Let's calculate anaesthesia time using the following formula:

Total Anesthesia Units=Base Units+Time Units+Modifying Units

For this example, let's assume:

- **Procedure**: Total pacemaker insertion
- **Base Units for the procedure**: 7 (based on the ASA relative value guide)
- **Anaesthesia start time**: 8:00 AM
- **Anaesthesia end time**: 10:15 AM
- **Physical Status Modifier**: P3 (Patient with severe systemic disease), which adds 3 units
- **Emergency Modifier**: ET (Emergency condition), which adds 2 units

Steps to Calculate

1. **Determine Anaesthesia Time**: Start time: 8:00 AM. End time: 10:15 AM. Total time: 2 hours and 15 minutes

2. **Convert Time to Units**: Time is typically billed in 15-minute increments. 2 hours and 15 minutes = 135 minutes.

3. **Number of 15-minute increments in 135 minutes** = 135 / 15 = 9 units

4. **Add Base Units**: Base units for the procedure = 7 units.

5. **Add Physical Status and Modifying Units**: Physical status modifier (P3) adds 3 units. Emergency modifier (ET) adds 2 units.

6. **Calculate Total Anesthesia Units**: Base Units: 7. Time Units: 9 Physical Status Units: 3 Emergency Units: 2

Total Anaesthesia Units=7+9+3+2=21

Physical Status Modifiers (P1-P6):

- **P1**: Normal healthy patient.
- **P2**: Patient with mild systemic disease.
- **P3**: Patient with severe systemic disease.
- **P4**: Patient with severe systemic disease that is a constant threat to life.
- **P5**: Moribund patient not expected to survive without the operation.
- **P6**: Declared brain-dead patient whose organs are being removed for donor purposes.

Modifiers for Anaesthesia Services:

- **AA**: Anaesthesia services performed personally by an anaesthesiologist.

- **AD**: Medical supervision by a physician for more than four concurrent anaesthesia procedures.
- **QK**: Medical direction of two to four concurrent anaesthesia procedures involving qualified individuals.
- **QX**: CRNA service with medical direction by a physician.
- **QZ**: CRNA service without medical direction by a physician.
- **QS**: Monitored anaesthesia care services.

Qualifying Circumstances Codes (99100-99140):

- Additional codes for extreme age, total body hypothermia, controlled hypotension, and emergency conditions.
- **99100**: Anaesthesia for patient of extreme age.
- **99116**: Anaesthesia complicated by utilization of total body hypothermia.
- **99135**: Anaesthesia complicated by utilization of controlled hypotension.
- **99140**: Anaesthesia complicated by emergency conditions.

ANAESTHESIA QUIZ

1. A 62-year-old patient with stable angina undergoes a total knee replacement under general anaesthesia. The anaesthesiologist administers anaesthesia and monitors the patient's cardiac status. Which CPT code and physical status modifier are appropriate?

   A) 01400, P1
   B) 01402, P2
   C) 01402, P3
   D) 01404, P2

2. An anaesthesiologist provides anaesthesia for a 45-year-old patient undergoing a radical nephrectomy due to renal cancer. The procedure lasts for 3.5 hours. Which CPT code should be used?

   A) 00862
   B) 00864
   C) 00865
   D) 00868

3. During a 2-hour surgical procedure for lumbar spine decompression, a 50-year-old patient with controlled diabetes receives epidural anaesthesia. Which anaesthesia code is most appropriate?

   A) 00630
   B) 00635
   C) 00620
   D) 00625

4. A 70-year-old patient with severe emphysema requires a thoracotomy to remove a lung mass. The anaesthesiologist

provides general anaesthesia. Which CPT code and physical status modifier should be reported?

A) 00540, P4
B) 00541, P3
C) 00546, P4
D) 00548, P5

5. A CRNA, directed by an anaesthesiologist, administers anaesthesia for a caesarean delivery on a healthy 28-year-old patient. Which anaesthesia code and modifier should be reported?

A) 01960, -QY
B) 01961, -QX
C) 01960, -QX
D) 01961, -QZ

6. A 35-year-old patient with a BMI of 40 is undergoing laparoscopic gastric bypass surgery. The anaesthesiologist provides general anaesthesia and monitors for potential complications due to obesity. Which anaesthesia code is appropriate?

A) 00797
B) 00842
C) 00840
D) 00796

7. During a 4-hour procedure to repair an aortic aneurysm, a 67-year-old patient with chronic kidney disease receives general anaesthesia. Which CPT code and physical status modifier are appropriate?

A) 00562, P4
C) 00566, P3
C) 00567, P4
D) 00568, P5

ANSWER KEY

1. **C) 01402, P3**

   Explanation: CPT code 01402 is for anaesthesia during total knee replacement with a physical status modifier P3 for a patient with severe systemic disease like stable angina.

2. **A) 00862**

   Explanation: CPT code 00862 is appropriate for anaesthesia during a radical nephrectomy, a procedure involving the kidney.

3. **B) 00635**

   CPT code 00635 is used for anaesthesia during procedures involving the lumbar spine, including decompression.

4. **C) 00546, P4**

   Explanation: CPT code 00546 is for anaesthesia during a thoracotomy, and modifier P4 indicates a patient with a severe systemic disease like emphysema.

5. **C) 01960, -QX**

   Explanation: CPT code 01960 is used for anaesthesia during a caesarean delivery, with modifier -QX for CRNA services under anaesthesiologist direction.

6. **A) 00797**

   Explanation: CPT code 00797 is used for anaesthesia during laparoscopic bariatric surgery, such as a gastric bypass.

7. **A) 00562, P4**

   Explanation: CPT code 00562 is for anaesthesia during an aortic aneurysm repair, with P4 for a patient with severe systemic disease like chronic kidney disease.

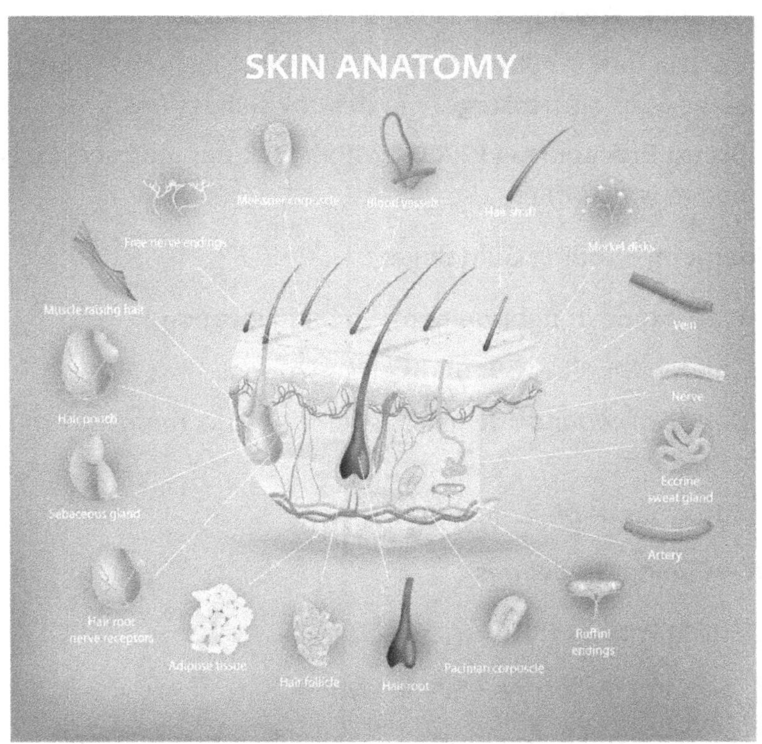

Anatomical Sites

- The integumentary system covers skin and subcutaneous tissues, including nails and breast.
- Codes are often specific to the anatomical site of the procedure.

Categories of Procedure

- **Incision and Drainage (10040-10180)**: Includes abscesses, cysts, hematomas, seromas, and other fluid collections.
- **Debridement (11000-11047)**: Removal of dead, damaged, or infected tissue to improve healing potential.
- **Excision—Benign and Malignant Lesions (11400-11646)**: Removal of tumours, cysts, and other lesions.
- **Repair—Simple, Intermediate, and Complex (12001-13160)**: Suturing of wounds, including layered closures.
- **Destruction (17000-17286)**: Procedures like cryosurgery, laser surgery, or electrosurgery to destroy skin lesions.
- **Breast Procedures (19000-19499)**: Includes biopsies, excisions, and mastectomies.

Debridement – Coding Guidelines

i. Watch type of debridement, size and location.

ii. Append Modifier 59 for different wounds.

iii. Depth of wound (deepest level of tissue removed) must be coded first.

iv. Add wounds of same depth.

Repair – Coding Guidelines

i. Which type of closure?

    a. Simple closure – Single layer.

    b. Intermediate closure – Layered closure / simple closure with heavy contamination.

    c. Complex – More than layered.

ii. Location on the body.

iii. **Add repairs** on the same type and body area.

iv. Sequence the most severe first.

v. Add modifier 59 for different subsequent repairs.

Adjacent Tissue Transfer (ATT)

- Code according to the location on the body.

- Code according to the size of different defects.

- Excision codes are bundled with ATT codes.

- Simple repairs are bundled.

- Intermediate and complex repairs can be reported separately.

Skin Replacement Surgery – Surgical / Wound Preparation

i. Code according to the location in the body.

ii. Code according to the size.

iii. Add the surface area of the wound from the same anatomical location.

iv. Modifier 59 for different wounds.

v. Under certain circumstances, complex closure and ATT can be combined.

Skin Grafts

It is divided into two:

i. Autograft – It comes from patient.

    a. Split thickness autograft

    b. Full thickness autograft

ii. Skin substitute grafts – It didn't come from patient.

    a. Allograft / Homograft – Same species / Different person

    b. Xenograft – Different species (animal)

    c. Artificial skin brands (Integra, Dermagraft, Dermabond)

Coding Guidelines

i. Wound preparation at the time of graft? (Code it)

ii. Type of graft?

iii. Thickness? (full thickness, split thickness)

iv. Code according to location on the body

v. Debridement bundled UNLESS prolonged cleansing (separate procedure)

vi. No modifier 59 on graft. But do code it on wound preparation.

Flaps (Coding Guidelines)

i. Code the formation (creating)

ii. Code the delay (cutting off an extended or delayed period of time)

iii. Code the transfer (attaching it to the recipient site)

iv. Code the skin grafts and donor site separately.

v. Code separate immobilization devices (casts or straps)

Burn Codes – Coding Guidelines

i. Code as per percentage of body area burnt.

ii. Depth of burn.

iii. Dressings are bundled.

MOHS Microscopic Surgery

Mohs surgery is often performed in stages, with each stage involving the removal of tissue and subsequent examination under a microscope. Coding is based on the number of stages completed during the surgery. **Example:** If a surgeon performs three stages of Mohs surgery to remove all cancerous tissue, you would code for three stages. Each additional stage beyond the first one is coded separately.

i.   Code according to location in the body.

ii.   First stage (17311 – 17313) – First slice only upto 5 block bundles

iii.   Each additional stage (17312-17314) have upto 5 bundles

iv.   Additional blocks are coded (each separately) with an add-on code (17315)

v.   Code Repairs / ATT / Grafts additionally.

vi.   Code Biopsy ONLY if diagnosed during same encounter as Moh's procedure with Modifier 59.

vii.   DO NOT code pathology for Moh's procedure.

INTEGUMENTARY SYSTEM QUIZ

1. A patient undergoes excision of a 1.5 cm benign lesion from the back and a 2.5 cm malignant lesion from the face during the same session. Which codes and modifiers should be reported?

   A) 11402, 11622
   B) 11402, 11622-59
   C) 11402-59, 11622
   D) 11402, 11622-51

2. When coding for wound debridement, if multiple wounds are treated at the same depth but at different anatomical sites, what is the appropriate coding practice?

   A) Use one code for all wounds
   B) Code each wound separately with modifier 59
   C) Code the largest wound only
   D) Bundle all wounds under a single code

3. A patient has a 10% total body surface area (TBSA) burn involving both second and third-degree burns. Which factor is crucial when coding the burn?

   A) The depth of the burn
   B) The percentage of the burn
   C) The type of dressing used
   D) The location of the burn

4. During a Mohs surgery, the surgeon performs three stages on the cheek, with six tissue blocks examined in the second stage. Which codes should be used?

   A) 17311, 17312
   B) 17311, 17312, 17315
   C) 17311, 17312, 17312-59
   D) 17311, 17315

5. A 2.0 cm malignant lesion is excised from the patient's left upper arm, with a 0.5 cm margin. What is the correct CPT code for this procedure?

    A) 11402
    B) 11404
    C) 11602
    D) 11604

6. A surgeon performs an adjacent tissue transfer (ATT) of 15 sq cm on the trunk and excises a 2.0 cm benign lesion from the back during the same procedure. How should this be coded?

    A) 14301, 11402
    B) 14001, 11402
    C) 14301, 11402-59
    D) 14001, 11402-51

7. For skin grafting, how should the graft be coded when an autograft is taken from the patient's thigh and applied to a wound on the arm?

    A) Code only the application site
    B) Code both the donor and recipient sites
    C) Code the donor site only
    D) Code the recipient site and add modifier 59

8. A patient with a history of keloid scars undergoes destruction of multiple pre-malignant lesions using cryotherapy. How should the destruction of these lesions be coded?

    A) 17000 for the first lesion, 17003 for each additional
    B) 17003 for each lesion
    C) 17000 for each lesion
    D) 17004 for all lesions combined

9. A patient with a dystrophic nail condition requires the trimming of all ten toenails. Which HCPCS Level II code should be used?

   A) G0127
   B) G0168
   C) G0295
   D) 11720

10. When performing a complex closure on the cheek involving layered closure, which factor does NOT affect the choice of CPT code?

    A) The length of the wound
    B) The number of layers closed
    C) The location of the wound
    D) The type of suture material used

ANSWER KEY

1. **B) 11402, 11622-59**

    Explanation: The code 11402 is for the excision of the benign lesion, and 11622 is for the excision of the malignant lesion. Modifier 59 is used to indicate that these are separate procedures.

2. **B) Code each wound separately with modifier 59**

    Explanation: When debridement is performed on wounds at the same depth but different anatomical sites, each wound should be coded separately with modifier 59 to indicate distinct services.

3. **A) The depth of the burn**

    Explanation: When coding burns, the depth (second or third degree) is crucial in determining the correct code, along with the percentage of the body area affected.

4. **B) 17311, 17312, 17315**

    Explanation: 17311 is used for the first stage, 17312 for the second stage, and 17315 for the additional tissue blocks examined in the second stage.

5. **C) 11602**

    Explanation: Code 11602 is used for the excision of malignant skin lesions on the arm, measuring 1.1 to 2.0 cm in diameter, including margins.

6. **C) 14301, 11402-59**

    Explanation: Code 14301 is for the ATT on the trunk, and 11402 is for the excision of the benign lesion. Modifier 59 is used to indicate that these are distinct procedures.

7. **B) Code both the donor and recipient sites**

    Explanation: When skin grafting is performed, both the donor site (thigh) and the recipient site (arm) should be coded separately.

8. **A) 17000 for the first lesion, 17003 for each additional**

    Explanation: Code 17000 is used for the destruction of the first pre-malignant lesion, and 17003 is used for each additional lesion destroyed.

9. **A) G0127**

    Explanation: HCPCS Level II code G0127 is used for the trimming of dystrophic nails, any number, for Medicare patients.

10. **D) The type of suture material used**

    Explanation: The choice of CPT code for a complex closure is based on the location, length of the wound, and the number of layers closed, not on the suture material used.

Chapter 4

Musculoskeletal System – Coding Guidelines (20000 Series)

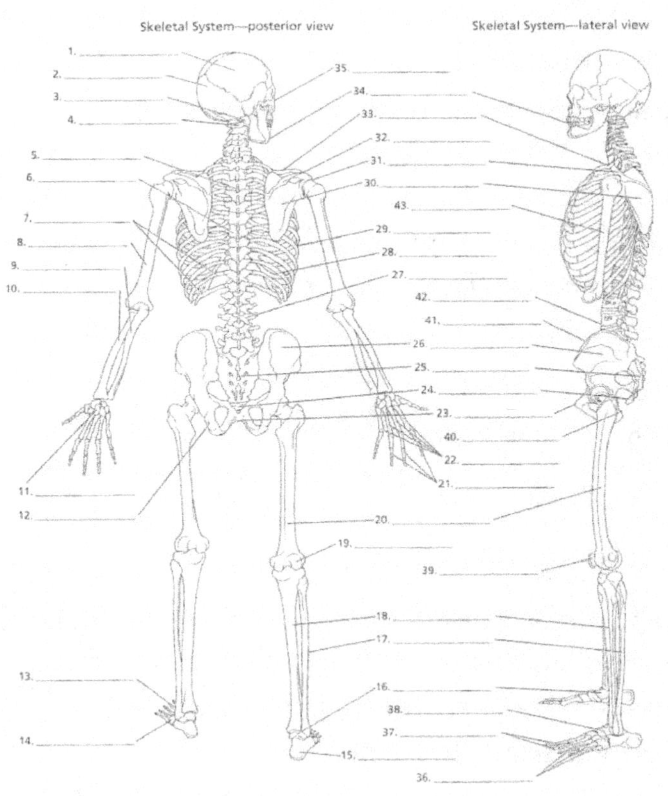

    i.   C – Cervical

    ii.   T – Thoracic

    iii.   L – Lumbar

    iv.   S – Sacral

HCPCS Level II

Orthotic and Prosthetics

Basic Orthopaedic Supplies

- o   Crutches
- o   Canes Walker
- o   Traction Devices
- o   Wheelchair & other orthopaedic supplies

Modifiers

    i.   50 – Bilateral

    ii.   59 – Distinct Procedure

    iii.   RT – Right

    iv.   LT – Left

    v.   FA – F9 – Specific Fingers

    vi.   TA – T9 – Specific Toes

Coding Guidelines (20100 – 20103)

    i.   Keep a note on keywords like gunshot wound, stabbing, deep wound exploration, enlargement, debridement etc.

    ii.   Watch bundled codes for example debridement, ligation or coagulation of MINOR blood vessels.

    iii.   DO NOT report repair and debridement codes with code range 20100-20103.

iv. DO NOT use codes ranging from (20100-20103) if Thoracotomy or Laparotomy is performed with bundled items or repairs.

v. Repair of major structures or major blood vessels requiring laparotomy / thoracotomy - Code for that system.

vi. If ONLY Minor skin repair is done NO EXPLORATION, code from the Integumentary System.

Trigger Point Injections – Coding Guidelines

i. Are we injecting muscles or joints? Number of Muscles?

ii. Watch the type of joint (small, medium, large)?

iii. NOT CODED According to number of injections

Halo, Pins, Implants & Fixation Devices – Coding Guidelines

i. Watch the type of instrumentation

ii. Implant vs Pins

iii. Uni plane means pins line up on one plane

iv. Multi plane means pins line up on multiple plane

Fracture Code Guidelines

i. Type

    a. Open

    b. Closed

    c. Percutaneous

    d. Any manipulation done?

ii. If the fracture is not documented code it as CLOSED

iii. Initial casts and removals are bundled in initial code.

Keywords For Fracture

i.   Open Fracture: Internal fixation, Intramedullary rod, Open reduction, Surgical opening of the fracture.

ii. Closed Treatment: No fixation, With or without manipulation, Cast application, Closed reduction.

iii. Percutaneous Treatment: External Fixation, Skeletal Fixation, Traction, Pins, Wires.

Arthrodesis Coding Guidelines

i.   Which approach? Code as per the approach used; lateral, anterior, posterior, spinal deformity

ii. Which instrumentation? Codes will be selected on the type of instrumentation; anterior vs posterior, segmental vs non-segmental.

iii. The number of spaces. Determine the number of levels.

iv. Code for bone grafts – Check if it is an allograft, autograft, morselized vs structural graft. Then use the appropriate codes.

v.   Do not use modifier 51 and 62 with instrumentation and grafting. In graft and instrumentation codes if modifier 51 and 62 are used, you may eliminate the option choices.

vi. Certain nervous system procedures, for example, discectomy, corpectomy can be used with arthrodesis codes but modifier 51 must be used.

Instrumentation Coding Guidelines

i.   Segmental Instrumentation – Attachment at each end of repair area and at least one other attachments in the area being repaired.

ii. Non-Segmental Instrumentation – Attachment of device at each end of the area being repaired.

Other Important Coding Tips

i. Tumour Excision – Check if the tumour excision is intramuscular or subcutaneous and code accordingly. Simple and intermediate repair is bundled in tumour excision, no need to code it separately.

ii. While coding for biopsy, check if the biopsy is for bone or muscle. Check if it is a superficial biopsy or a deep biopsy, open biopsy or percutaneous, choose codes accordingly.

iii. Code 29880 vs 29881 – 29880 - Arthroscopy with meniscectomy (medial AND lateral). 29881- Arthroscopy with meniscectomy (medial OR lateral).

iv. Code 29875 vs 29885 – In this code the keyword is drilling however, in 29885 – Along with drilling, bone graft will be used.

MUSCULOSKELETAL SYSTEM – QUIZ

1. A surgeon performs an open reduction and internal fixation (ORIF) of a comminuted fracture of the right femoral shaft. During the same surgery, a separate incision is made to treat a closed fracture of the left distal tibia with a percutaneous pinning. Which codes and modifiers should be reported?

   A) 27507-RT, 27758-LT
   B) 27507-50, 27758-59
   C) 27506-LT, 27758-RT
   D) 27506-RT, 27758-LT-59

2. A patient presents with bilateral carpal tunnel syndrome. The surgeon performs a release on the right wrist during one session and plans to perform the left wrist release in a future session. How should this be coded for the current procedure?

   A) 64721-LT
   B) 64721-RT
   C) 64721-50
   D) 64721-RT, 64721-59

3. A surgeon performs a total knee arthroplasty on the right knee, and during the same procedure, performs an arthroscopic meniscectomy on the left knee. Which of the following is the correct coding and use of modifiers?

   A) 27447-RT, 29881-LT-59
   B) 27447-LT, 29881-RT-51
   C) 27447-50, 29881-59
   D) 27447-RT, 29881-LT

4. During a single operative session, a surgeon performs a lumbar spinal fusion at L3-L5 with posterior segmental instrumentation. Which codes and modifiers should be used?

A) 22612, 22842
B) 22612-51, 22842-RT
C) 22612-RT, 22842-LT
D) 22612, 22842-59

5. A patient undergoes a closed treatment of a percutaneous fracture of the left fibula with external fixation. What is the correct coding and modifier application?

A) 27792-LT
B) 27792-RT
C) 27793-LT
D) 27792-LT-59

6. A physician performs a percutaneous needle biopsy of the right femur. During the same session, a bone biopsy of the left humerus is also performed. What is the correct way to code these procedures?

A) 20225-RT, 20225-LT-59
B) 20225-50
C) 20220-RT, 20220-LT-59
D) 20225-RT, 20225-LT

7. A patient receives an arthroscopic chondroplasty of the right knee and a separate partial meniscectomy of the same knee during the same operative session. How should this be coded?

A) 29877-RT, 29881-RT-59
B) 29881-RT, 29877-RT
C) 29877-50, 29881-50
D) 29881-RT-59, 29877-RT

8. A surgeon performs a closed treatment of a right humeral shaft fracture with manipulation. Later in the same session, the left clavicle is surgically repaired due to a separate injury. What is the correct coding and modifier usage?

    A) 23615-RT, 24505-LT-59
    B) 23615-LT, 24505-RT-59
    C) 24505-RT, 23615-LT
    D) 24505-50, 23615-50

9. A surgeon performs an arthroscopic rotator cuff repair on the left shoulder, and in the same session, removes a loose body from the right elbow joint arthroscopically. What is the correct coding and use of modifiers?

    A) 29827-RT, 29834-LT
    B) 29827-LT, 29834-RT-59
    C) 29827-50, 29834-59
    D) 29827-LT, 29834-59

10. A patient with osteoarthritis undergoes total hip arthroplasty on the right hip. A few weeks later, the left hip is also replaced. How should these procedures be coded?

    A) 27130-RT, 27132-59
    B) 27130-LT, 27130-RT
    C) 27132-LT, 27130-RT
    D) 27130-RT, 27130-LT

KEY ANSWERS

1. **D) 27506-RT, 27758-LT-59**

   Explanation: Code 27506 is for ORIF of the femoral shaft, and 27758 is for percutaneous skeletal fixation of a tibial fracture. Modifiers RT and LT indicate the sides, and modifier 59 is used to signify a distinct procedural service.

2. **B) 64721-RT**

   Explanation: Code 64721 is for carpal tunnel release, and modifier RT indicates the right wrist. Since the left wrist will be treated in a separate session, no need for bilateral (50) or distinct procedure (59) modifiers.

3. **A) 27447-RT, 29881-LT-59**

   Explanation: Code 27447 is for total knee arthroplasty, and 29881 is for arthroscopic meniscectomy. Modifiers RT and LT denote the sides, while modifier 59 indicates the meniscectomy was a distinct procedural service on a different knee.

4. **A) 22612, 22842**

   Explanation: Code 22612 is for lumbar spinal fusion, and 22842 is for posterior segmental instrumentation. Both are reported separately without the need for modifiers since they represent distinct services in the same operative session.

5. **A) 27792-LT**

   Explanation: Code 27792 is for closed treatment of a percutaneous fracture with external fixation, and modifier LT indicates the left fibula. Modifier 59 is unnecessary as no separate, distinct procedure is performed.

6. **A) 20225-RT, 20225-LT-59**

   Explanation: Code 20225 is for a bone biopsy. Modifiers RT and LT indicate the side-specific procedures, and modifier 59 is used to signify the procedures were distinct from one another.

7. **A) 29877-RT, 29881-RT-59**

   Explanation: Code 29877 is for chondroplasty, and 29881 is for meniscectomy. Modifier RT indicates the right knee, and modifier 59 is used to indicate the meniscectomy was a separate and distinct procedure.

8. **A) 23615-RT, 24505-LT-59**

   Explanation: Code 24505 is for the closed treatment of a humeral fracture with manipulation, and 23615 is for the surgical repair of the clavicle. Modifiers RT and LT indicate the sides, and modifier 59 is used to indicate that these are distinct procedures.

9. **B) 29827-LT, 29834-RT-59**

   Explanation: Code 29827 is for arthroscopic rotator cuff repair, and 29834 is for the removal of a loose body. Modifiers LT and RT indicate the specific sides, and modifier 59 is used to indicate a distinct procedural service.

10. **D) 27130-RT, 27130-LT**

    Explanation: Code 27130 is for total hip arthroplasty. Since the procedures were performed at different times, the correct coding includes 27130-RT for the right hip and 27130-LT for the left hip without any need for additional modifiers.

Respiratory & Cardiovascular System - CPC Coding Guidelines (30000)

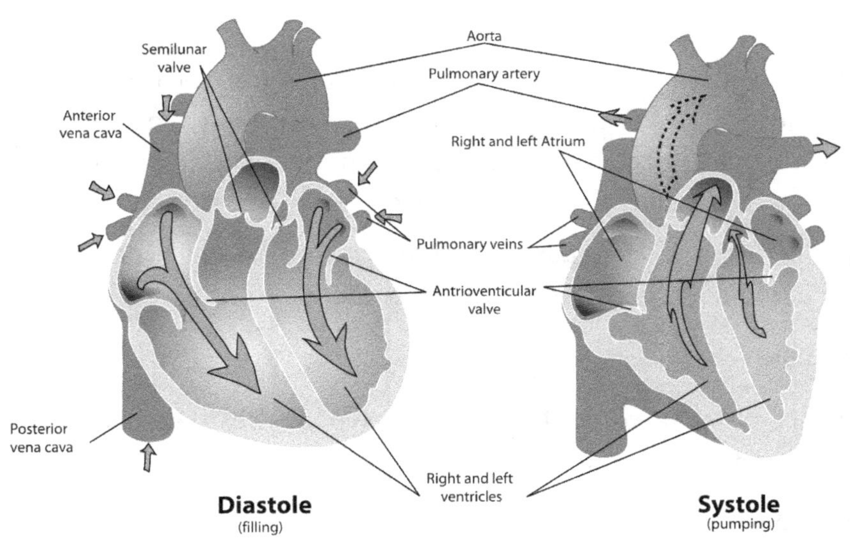

Anatomical Understanding

i. Respiratory System Components - Nose, sinuses, larynx, trachea, bronchi, lungs, and pleura. Code as per the anatomical locations.

ii. Procedures Covered - Includes diagnostic and therapeutic procedures like endoscopies, biopsies, and surgeries. Code as per the procedure performed.

Commonly Used Modifiers for Respiratory & Cardiovascular System

- **Modifier 50**: Bilateral procedure.
- **Modifier 51**: Multiple procedures.
- **Modifier 52**: Reduced services.
- **Modifier 53**: Discontinued procedure.
- **Modifier 59**: Distinct procedural service.
- **Modifier 76**: Repeat procedure by the same physician.
- **Modifier 77**: Repeat procedure by another physician.

Bundling Rules

i. Diagnostic procedure is always a part of surgical procedure, do not code diagnostic procedure separately, code for only surgical procedure. When just diagnosis is performed then one can code diagnostic procedure codes separately.

ii. In rhinoplasty (nose job), skin closure or repair codes are bundled, do not code them separately.

Pacemaker

The pacemaker *sends electrical pulses to your heart to keep it beating regularly and not too slowly.*

Pacemaker (Terminologies)

i. Pulse Generator (Battery)

ii. Electrodes (wire or leads) Leads describe the type of pacemaker.

iii. Transvenous (Through the vein)

Pacemaker – Coding Guidelines

i. If document doesn't specify whether the pacemaker / defibrillator is permanent or temporary, code it as permanent.

ii. Insertion of pacemaker / defibrillator is first time or not – by default it is first or initial insertion.

iii. What are you coding for – Pacemaker / defibrillator / battery / leads / leadless system. Then code accordingly.

iv. Type of pacemaker – Temporary / permanent. It is important to decide the type of pacemaker and then code accordingly.

v. How are these leads implanted – transvenous or through chest or multiple chamber (biventricular).

vi. If skin pocket was created or not – skin pocket creation or revision is bundled in the system.

vii. Check if the pacemaker is single or dual chambered and then select the appropriate codes.

Catheter Placement – Coding Guidelines

In catheter placement, check for veins in the given scenario, which vein is used? Central vein or peripheral vein.

i. **Keywords for central vein are:** Subclavian vein, jugular vein, femoral vein, inferior vena cava. Any one of these will be mentioned in the question.

Central vein can be tunnelled or non-tunnelled. Sometimes, it is mentioned in the question, if the vein is tunnelled or non-tunnelled. If it is not mentioned then look for the keywords.

In tunnelled there is **chest incision and tunnel creation**. Whereas in non-tunnelled there **is direct puncture of the central vein.**

i. **Keywords for peripheral vein are:** basilic, cephalic, saphenous.

ii. Further check for pump, port, age of the patient, if catheter only is used or catheter and pump is used or catheter or port is used and accordingly select the codes.

Coronary Artery Bypass Graft (CABG) – Coding Guidelines

   i. First check which type of graft is harvested? Venous graft, arterial graft or combined graft.

  ii. Venous graft code ranges from 33510-33516. **We do not use arterial graft codes ranging from (33533 -33536) with venous graft.** Vein included are brachial vein, ulnar vein, cephalic vein, basilic vein, brachiocephalic vein, subclavian vein.

 iii. Combined graft code ranges from (33517-33522). **In this case we code the arterial graft codes first (33533-33536).**

 iv. For arterial graft codes range from (33533-33536).

  v. For saphenous vein, mammary and lower extremity artery harvesting, no separate codes are required. These are bundled codes.

 vi. Endoscopy codes can be coded only with code range 33510 – 33523.

vii. No co-surgeon modifiers for harvest code use only assistant surgeon modifiers.

QUIZ

1. A 65-year-old patient with a history of coronary artery disease undergoes a combined coronary artery bypass grafting (CABG) procedure. The surgeon harvests both the saphenous vein and the internal mammary artery, creating a single arterial graft and two venous grafts. Which of the following is the correct coding sequence for this procedure?

   A) 33534, 33517
   B) 33510, 33533
   C) 33512, 33535 – 51
   D) 33518, 33533

2. A surgeon performs a diagnostic bronchoscopy on a patient with suspected lung cancer, followed by a therapeutic bronchoalveolar lavage (BAL) and a transbronchial biopsy of the left lower lobe during the same session. How should this be coded?

   A) 31628, 31624-51, 31622-59
   B) 31622, 31628-51, 31624-51
   C) 31628, 31624-51
   D) 31622, 31624-51, 31628-59

3. A patient undergoes the insertion of a permanent biventricular pacemaker with transvenous placement of two leads: one in the right atrium and one in the right ventricle. Later, due to complications, the physician revises the skin pocket and replaces the pulse generator. How should these procedures be coded?

   A) 33208, 33228-76
   B) 33208, 33216-59
   C) 33225, 33228
   D) 33208, 33228-78

4. A patient presents with severe chronic obstructive pulmonary disease (COPD) and undergoes a right and left lung biopsy via bronchoscopy. The procedure is completed without complications. Which code(s) and modifier(s) should be used for accurate reporting?

    A) 31628, 31632-50
    B) 31625, 31628-50
    C) 31628, 31632
    D) 31628-50

5. A patient undergoes catheter placement into the subclavian vein for central venous access. The catheter is tunneled, and a subcutaneous port is placed. The patient is 45 years old. Which of the following codes best represents this procedure?

    A) 36558
    B) 36561
    C) 36560
    D) 36565

6. A 70-year-old patient requires the removal and replacement of a permanent pacemaker generator, with the leads left intact. The procedure is complicated by a wound infection that necessitates extensive debridement and irrigation. Which of the following coding sequences is correct?

    A) 33227, 33216-51, 11043-59
    B) 33228, 11044-59
    C) 33228, 33233-51, 11044-59
    D) 33227, 33208-51, 11044-59

7. A patient has a history of severe mitral valve stenosis and undergoes an open mitral valve replacement with the insertion of a transvenous pacemaker lead into the right ventricle. The

pacemaker was previously placed but only had atrial leads. Which is the correct code sequence?

A) 33430, 33208
B) 33430, 33207
C) 33425, 33207
D) 33430, 33216

8. A 58-year-old patient undergoes a bilateral diagnostic bronchoscopy followed by the removal of two foreign bodies, one from each lung. Which code and modifier combination should be used?

A) 31635-50
B) 31622, 31635-51
C) 31635, 31635-59
D) 31635-50, 31635-51

9. A 45-year-old male patient undergoes a transvenous insertion of a single-lead pacemaker. The documentation does not specify whether it is temporary or permanent. What is the correct coding?

A) 33206
B) 33207
C) 33208
D) 33216

10. A thoracoscopic lung biopsy is performed on a patient with a mass in the right lower lobe, followed by a thoracoscopic lobectomy of the same lung. What is the correct coding sequence?

A) 32663, 32666-51
B) 32666-59, 32663
C) 32663, 32666-59
D) 32666

KEY ANSWERS

1. **D) 33518, 33533**

   Explanation: The correct coding for a combined graft procedure that includes one arterial graft (internal mammary artery) and multiple venous grafts (saphenous vein) is to use 33518 for the venous grafts and 33533 for the arterial graft. Modifier 51 is not necessary as these codes inherently indicate multiple procedures.

2. **C) 31628, 31624-51**

   Explanation: The diagnostic bronchoscopy (31622) is not coded separately as it is bundled into the therapeutic procedures. Code 31628 is for the transbronchial biopsy, and 31624 is for the bronchoalveolar lavage (BAL). Modifier 51 indicates multiple procedures performed during the same session.

3. **D) 33208, 33228-78**

   Explanation: Code 33208 is used for the initial insertion of a permanent dual-chamber pacemaker. The replacement of the pulse generator and revision of the skin pocket is coded as 33228 with modifier 78, indicating an unplanned return to the operating room for a related procedure during the postoperative period.

4. **D) 31628-50**

   Explanation: Code 31628 is for a transbronchial lung biopsy via bronchoscopy, and since both the right and left lungs were biopsied, modifier 50 (Bilateral procedure) should be used to indicate this.

5. **B) 36561**

   Explanation: Code 36561 is for the tunneled placement of a central venous catheter with a subcutaneous port for patients aged 5 years or older. The subclavian vein is a central vein, and the tunneling is indicated by this code.

6. **B) 33228, 11044-59**

   Explanation: Code 33228 is for the removal and replacement of the pacemaker pulse generator with leads left intact. The extensive debridement (11044) is coded separately with modifier 59 to indicate it as a distinct procedural service.

7. **D) 33430, 33216**

   Explanation: Code 33430 is for an open mitral valve replacement. Code 33216 is used for the insertion of a transvenous pacemaker lead into the right ventricle, complementing the previously placed atrial lead.

8. **A) 31635-50**

   Explanation: Code 31635 is used for bronchoscopy with the removal of a foreign body. Since the procedure is bilateral, modifier 50 should be applied. No need for additional codes as the diagnostic part is bundled with the therapeutic procedure.

9. **A) 33206**

   Explanation: Code 33206 is for the transvenous insertion of a permanent single-lead pacemaker. If the documentation doesn't specify whether it is temporary or permanent, it is typically assumed to be permanent unless otherwise stated.

10. **D) 32666**

    Explanation: Code 32666 is for a thoracoscopic lobectomy, which includes the biopsy as part of the procedure. The biopsy is bundled into the lobectomy code, so it should not be coded separately.

Chapter 6

Digestive System - Coding Guidelines (40000)

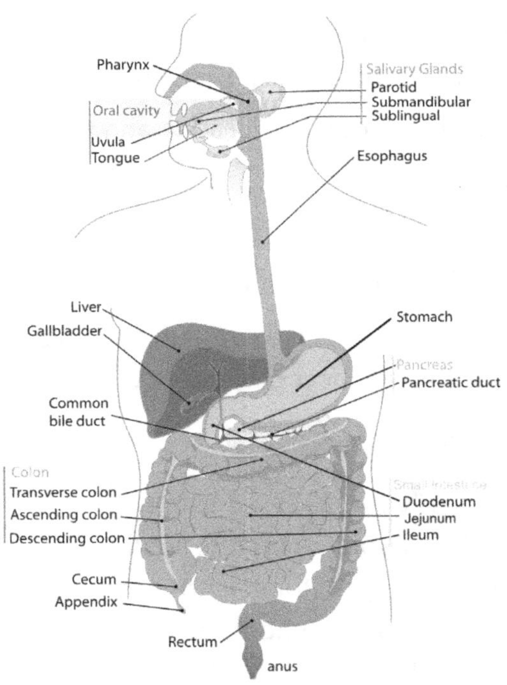

Important Suffix

The following suffixes are crucial, and students must thoroughly understand their precise meanings. Mastery of these suffixes will enable students to accurately select the correct codes.

i. Otomy – Means incision, making a cut

ii. Ectomy – This term denotes surgical removal, excision or resection.

iii. Ostomy – Means permanent opening.

iv. Krapny/Pexy/Plasty – Means repair.

v. Lysis – Means freeing up or destruction

vi. Ablation – Destruction

Digestive System Coding Guidelines

i. Diagnostic procedure is always a part of surgical procedure. When there is a surgical procedure followed by the diagnostic procedure, **code the surgical procedure only.**

ii. Code as per the anatomical location and the approach involved.

   i. Open procedure – incision, biopsy, excision, insertion / introduction, removal, repair.

   ii. Endoscopic – Use of scope through existing opening.

   iii. Laparoscopic – Usage of laparoscopic instruments for example ports, trocar placement etc.

Digestive System Procedures

Esophagoscopy (43200-43232) - Esophagoscopy is a medical procedure that allows your doctor to look inside your esophagus. This procedure helps your doctor diagnose conditions that affect your esophagus. It is done using an endoscope or esophagoscope, which is a thin tube with an attached light and camera.

In this procedure scope is passed through the esophagus. Scope may be advanced into stomach but do not cross pylorus.

Esophagogastroduodenoscopy (EGD) - EGD is a diagnostic endoscopic procedure used to visualize the oropharynx, esophagus, stomach and proximal duodenum.

Key points

Check things like dilation, with band ligation etc. in order to code appropriately.

Important Modifiers

i. Modifier 52 – If the service or procedure has been partially reduced or eliminated at the patient's discretion.

ii. Modifier 53 – Is used due to certain circumstance when a physician or other qualified health care professional elects to terminate a surgical or medical procedure.

Endoscopic Retrograde Cholangiopancreatography (ERCP)

It is an endoscopic procedure used to identify the presence of stones, tumor, or narrowing in the biliary and pancreatic ducts. After the endoscope is properly placed, a catheter is advanced which will inject a contrast agent through the ducts. If scope passes **beyond second portion of duodenum, becomes an ERCP** procedure.

Endoscopy Intestine (44360-44379)

When the scope passes beyond the second portion of duodenum and reaches jejunum or ileum, it becomes intestinal endoscopy. Other things to check before coding (removal of foreign body, biopsy etc.)

Appendectomy

Appendectomy is surgery to remove the appendix, which is usually found in the right lower side of the abdomen. Appendectomy is usually carried out on an emergency basis to treat appendicitis (inflamed appendix). A ruptured appendix can cause peritonitis, which is a potentially life-threatening complication.

If appendix is ruptured code 44960, if not ruptured code, 44950

Procedure Related Codes

i. **Proctosigmoidoscopy** – The code range is from 45300-45327, and anus, rectum and sigmoid colon is included.

ii. **Sigmoidoscopy** - The code range is from 45330-45346, and rectum and sigmoid colon and a pert of descending colon is included.

iii. **Colonoscopy** – The code range is from 45378-45398. is *a test to check inside your bowels*. This test can help find what's causing your bowel symptoms.

iv. **Tonsillectomy & Adnoidectomy** - Tonsils are small, round pieces of tissue located in the back of the mouth on both sides of the throat. Adenoids are similar to tonsils but located in back of the nasal cavity. Tonsils and adenoids are often removed when they become large and inflamed and begin to cause frequent infections. The procedure to remove tonsils is known as a **tonsillectomy**, and removal of the adenoids is called an **adenoidectomy**. Because they are often removed at the same time, the procedure is referred to as a tonsillectomy and adenoidectomy, or **T&A**. Do not append modifier 50 with tonsillectomy and adenoidectomy codes because these codes represents bilateral procedure. Use 52 modifier for unilateral procedure.

Hernia

It is a combination of pressure and an opening or weakness of muscle or fascia. The pressure pushes an organ or tissue through the opening or weak spot. Sometimes the muscle weakness is present at birth. But more often, it happens later in life.

Types of Hernia

i. Inguinal (inner groin)

ii. Femoral (outer groin)

   iii.   Incisional (resulting from incision)

   iv.   Umblical (belly button)

   v.   Hiatal (upper stomach)

Hernia Coding Tips

   i.   Check if hernia repair is open v/s laparoscopic.

   ii.   Type of hernia (inguinal / femoral / umbilical / incisional/ ventral)

   iii.   Age of the patient.

   iv.   Initial v/s recurrent.

   v.   Reducible (well defined v/s strangulated / incarcerated / obstructed).

Key Coding Guidelines

   i.   For obstructed hernia the implantation of mesh is BUNDLED.

   ii.   Only for incisional or ventral hernia, mesh implantation is reported separately.

   iii.   Esophagogastroduodenoscopy (EGD) describes the viewing of esophagus, stomach, and the duodenum. Whenever this procedure is performed, check all the anatomical locations are tested.

   iv.   Endoscopy allows moderate sedation to be coded additionally.

   v.   Modifier 59 is appended to the secondary procedure to indicate that the procedure was performed during a different operative session.

QUIZ

1. A patient undergoes a diagnostic esophagoscopy with biopsy of the esophagus. During the same session, the physician identifies a mass in the stomach and performs a biopsy through the same scope. Which of the following is the correct coding for this procedure?

   A) 43202, 43200-59
   B) 43202, 43239-59
   C) 43239, 43200-51
   D) 43200, 43202-59

2. A surgeon performs a laparoscopic inguinal hernia repair on a 50-year-old male. During the procedure, the hernia is found to be strangulated, and the surgeon implants a mesh. How should this procedure be coded?

   A) 49650, 49568
   B) 49507, 49585-22
   C) 49652
   D) 49521, 49568

3. A patient presents for a colonoscopy, during which a polypectomy is performed in the ascending colon. However, the procedure is terminated due to complications before reaching the transverse colon. Which of the following is the correct coding and modifier usage?

   A) 45385-53
   B) 45378-53, 45385
   C) 45378-52, 45385
   D) 45385-52

4. A 70-year-old patient undergoes a diagnostic ERCP, and during the procedure, a biliary stone is found and removed using a

basket. The endoscope reaches beyond the second portion of the duodenum. Which of the following codes and modifiers should be used?

A) 43262, 43264-59
B) 43264
C) 43260, 43262-51
D) 43262

5. A patient with chronic GERD undergoes an EGD with dilation of a stricture in the esophagus using a balloon. The procedure is successfully completed. What is the correct coding for this procedure?

A) 43235, 43248-51
B) 43235, 43220-52
C) 43248
D) 43220

6. A 45-year-old female patient undergoes a laparoscopic umbilical hernia repair with mesh implantation. The hernia was reducible. How should this be coded?

A) 49580, 49568
B) 49653, 49568
C) 49652
D) 49585

7. A patient undergoes a proctosigmoidoscopy with removal of a foreign body from the rectum. The procedure is performed under general anesthesia. Which of the following is the correct code?

A) 45303-59
B) 45330
C) 45307
D) 45300-51

8. A surgeon performs a laparoscopic repair of a recurrent incisional hernia with mesh implantation. What is the correct coding for this procedure?

    A) 49566, 49568
    B) 49656, 49568
    C) 49566
    D) 49656, 49568

9. A patient undergoes an appendectomy for a ruptured appendix with generalized peritonitis. The procedure is performed as an open surgery. Which of the following is the correct code?

    A) 44950
    B) 44960
    C) 44955
    D) 44970

10. During a diagnostic colonoscopy, the physician identifies a polyp in the sigmoid colon and removes it using cold biopsy forceps. Additionally, another polyp is found in the descending colon and removed via snare technique. How should this be coded?

    A) 45385, 45380-59
    B) 45380, 45385-51
    C) 45385, 45384-51
    D) 45378, 45385-59

KEY ANSWERS

1. **B) 43202, 43239-59**

   Explanation: Code 43202 is for esophagoscopy with biopsy, and 43239 is for EGD with biopsy. Since the scope was advanced from the esophagus to the stomach, modifier 59 should be appended to 43239 to indicate that a distinct procedure was performed in a different anatomical site during the same session.

2. **C) 49652**

   Explanation: Code 49652 is for laparoscopic repair of an inguinal hernia with strangulation. The mesh implantation is bundled with the code for strangulated or incarcerated hernia repair, so it should not be coded separately.

3. **A) 45385-53**

   Explanation: Code 45385 is for a colonoscopy with polypectomy. Modifier 53 is used to indicate that the procedure was terminated due to complications, as it signifies a discontinued procedure.

4. **B) 43264**

   Explanation: Code 43264 is for ERCP with removal of stones from the bile duct using a basket. Since the procedure is therapeutic and diagnostic, the diagnostic portion is included in the therapeutic code, so only 43264 is needed.

5. **C) 43248**

   Explanation: Code 43248 is for an EGD with dilation of an esophageal stricture using a balloon. The diagnostic EGD is bundled with the therapeutic dilation, so only 43248 is coded.

6. **C) 49652**

   Explanation: Code 49580 is for a laparoscopic umbilical hernia repair without mention of strangulation or incarceration. Mesh implantation (49568) is reported separately for reducible hernias as per coding guidelines.

7. **C) 45307**

   Explanation: Code 45307 is for a proctosigmoidoscopy with removal of a foreign body from the rectum. The use of general anesthesia is included in this code and does not require separate coding.

8. **B) 49656, 49568**

   Explanation: Code 49656 is for a laparoscopic repair of a recurrent incisional hernia, and 49568 is for the implantation of mesh. Mesh is reported separately in the case of incisional hernias.

9. **B) 44960**

   Explanation: Code 44960 is for an open appendectomy for a ruptured appendix with generalized peritonitis. This code includes the complexity of the procedure due to the rupture and peritonitis.

10. **A) 45385, 45380-59**

    Explanation: Code 45385 is for the removal of a polyp using a snare technique, and 45380 is for the removal of a polyp using cold biopsy forceps. Modifier 59 is appended to 45380 to indicate that the second polyp removal was a distinct procedure performed in a different anatomical site during the same session.

Chapter 7

Genito – Urinary System – Male and Female Reproductive System – Coding Guidelines (50000)

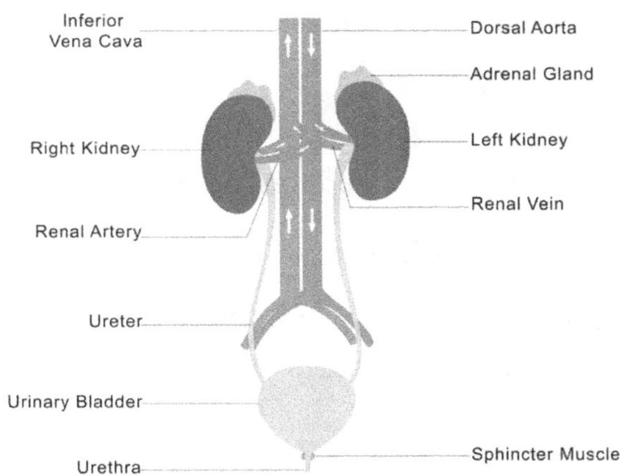

Common Terminologies and CPT Codes for Male Reproductive System

    i.   Incision – 54000 – 54015

    ii.   Destruction – 54050 – 54065

    iii.   Excision – 54100 – 54164

    iv.   Introduction – 54200 – 54250

    v.   Repair – 54300 – 54440

   vi.   Manipulation – 54450

Guidelines for Genitourinary Series

While checking the question, check what type of procedure it is, it will help in eliminating the wrong options:

    i.   Open

   ii.   Laparoscopic

  iii.   Endoscopic

Endoscopic Procedure in the Urinary System

    i.   Scout endoscopic procedure is a part of diagnostic and therapeutic procedure. DO NOT code them separately.

   ii.   Diagnostic endoscopy is always a part of therapeutic endoscopy.

  iii.   Multiple endoscopic procedures are appended by modifier 51

Other Urinary System Guidelines

    i.   In case of biopsy and excision in the same lesion, biopsy is not coded separately. Prostrate biopsy codes are: 55700, 55705, 55706

   ii.   Laparoscopic procedure is a part of surgical procedure and is not coded twice

  iii.   The insertion and removal of a temporary ureteral catheter (CPT 52005) during diagnostic or therapeutic cystourethroscopy / pyeloscopy is included in codes 52320-52356 and need not be coded separately.

  iv.   Stent insertion must be coded separately.

   v.   Colposcopy is a procedure to closely examine your cervix, vagina and vulva for signs of disease.

vi. Dilation of vagina (57400) and dilation of cervical canal (57800) is included in the respective procedure and need not be coded separately. Unless the code description specifically mentions, without cervical dilation.

i. **Nephrectomy** – Nephro is kidney and ectomy is removal. It is the procedure of removing kidney surgically.

    i. Open / Laparoscopic

    ii. Total nephrectomy (50220) / partial nephrectomy (50240) / laparoscopic nephrectomy (505543)

ii. **Nephrolithotomy** – Nephro is kidney, lith is stone, otomy is surgical opening, cutting into and removing something. It is removal of kidney stone by incision. Renal Calculi (kidney stone) and the procedure that breaks the stone into smaller pieces is called lithotripsy. Lith means stone and trip means to break. Code 50590 describes the use of lithotripsy wave machine, which sends shock waves to body from outside.

    i. Open incision (50060 – 50075)

    ii. Stone removal percutaneous; lithotripsy can be used for stone basket extraction – 50800

    iii. Percutaneous Lithotripsy – 50590

iii. **Kidney / Renal Transplant Coding Guidelines**

Renal transplant consists of 6 procedures

    i. Removal of kidney from cadaver

    ii. Removal of kidney from living donor

    iii. Cadaver donor backbench work

    iv. Living donor backbench work

    v. Additional reconstruction

    vi. Allotransplantation

Use modifier 51 for multiple procedure. Diagnostic scopes are bundled into the same surgical scope if not removed.

Circumcision (Extremely Important)

i. With clamp and ring block use 54150.

ii. Without clamp use 54160.

iii. Use modifier 52 with code 54150 when procedure is done without ring block.

iv. **Circumcision are of two types**

i. Topical (No Anaesthesia)

ii. Dorsal Penile Nerve Block

Coding Guideline

i. 54150 (Circumcision with clamp) CAN be used for neonates

ii. Use Modifier 52 (Reduced Services) WITHOUT dorsal penile nerve or ring nerve block.

v. **Prostrate Biopsy:**

Code range is from 55700-55706. Check for needle or punch vs incisional vs transperinial.

vi. **Vulvectomy**

A procedure to remove totally or partially vulva of a woman's outer genitals. Code range is from 55620 – 55640. There are different types of vulvectomy.

a. Simple – Removal of skin and superficial subcutaneous tissue.

b. Radical – Removal of skin and deep subcutaneous tissue.

c. Partial – Removal of less than 80% of vulvar area.

d. Complete – Removal of greater than 80% of vulvar area.

vii. **Hysterectomy**

It is a procedure to remove uterus. Before coding first check whether it is a/an

    a. Open / close / laparoscopic

    b. Check the procedure

    c. Abdominal v/s vaginal

    d. Partial v/s total

    e. Removal of ovary(s) and / or tube(s): Yes / No

        i. **Abdominal Hysterectomy:** If the uterus is removed through abdomen. (58150)

        ii. **Vaginal Hysterectomy:** If the uterus is removed from the vagina. (58152)

        iii. **Supracervical Hysterectomy:** It is a procedure to remove the uterus and not the cervix and the fallopian tube. (58180)

viii. **In Vitro Fertilization (IVF)**

Code ranges from 58970 – 58976. Check in the question what is being asked and only then code.

    i. 58970 – Follicle puncture for oocyte retrieval, any method.

    ii. 58974 – Embryo transfer, intrauterine

    iii. 58976 – Gamete, zygote, or embryo intrafallopian transfer, any method

(For laparoscopic adnexal procedures, see 58660-58673)

ix. **Vaginal Delivery, Antepartum and Postpartum Care**

    i. 59400 – Routine obstetric care including antepartum care, vaginal delivery (with or without episiotomy, and /

or forceps) and postpartum care. It is a full code. Use only when all these services are mentioned in the question. Delivery codes must be once but one can deliver multiple kids.

ii.   54909-59430 – Are separate codes, wherein the patient gets different services from different hospitals.

x.   **Abortion**

Abortion code ranges from 59812 – 59857. Abortion are of two types, while coding for abortion check the type of abortion.

1. Induced abortion

i.   Dilation and curettage

ii.   Dilation and evacuation

2. Spontaneous abortion

xi.   Complete abortion – The uterus is completely empty

xii.   Incomplete abortion – Uterus is partially empty

xiii.   Missed abortion – No symptoms but the heartbeat of the fetes is missing (fetes is dead)

QUIZ

1. A patient undergoes a total nephrectomy for a renal tumor via an open surgical approach. During the same session, the surgeon also performs a cystoscopy with ureteral stent insertion. How should these procedures be coded?

   A) 50220, 52005
   B) 50590, 52332-51
   C) 50220, 52332-51
   D) 50220, 52332

2. A surgeon performs a laparoscopic partial nephrectomy followed by a percutaneous lithotripsy on the same kidney during the same session. Which coding and modifier combination is correct?

   A) 50543, 50590-51
   B) 50590, 50543-51
   C) 50590, 50075-51
   D) 50543, 50075-51

3. During a cystourethroscopy, the surgeon performs a biopsy of a bladder lesion and then excises the lesion. Which CPT code(s) should be reported?

   A) 52354
   B) 52204, 52355-51
   C) 52224, 52204-51
   D) 52355

4. A laparoscopic-assisted vaginal hysterectomy (LAVH) with bilateral salpingo-oophorectomy is performed. Which code accurately reflects this procedure, and what factors should be considered in its selection?

A) 58150
B) 58552
C) 58180
D) 58152

5. A diagnostic cystourethroscopy is followed by therapeutic cystourethroscopy with stent insertion and lithotripsy. How should these procedures be coded?

A) 52005, 52320-51, 52332-51
B) 52320, 52332-51
C) 52332-51, 50590
D) 52320, 52005

6. A patient undergoes a partial vulvectomy involving less than 80% of the vulva, including both superficial and deep subcutaneous tissue. Which CPT code is most appropriate?

A) 56630
B) 56620
C) 56625
D) 56640

7. During a vaginal delivery, the patient requires an episiotomy and the use of forceps. The provider also handles antepartum and postpartum care. Which code should be reported for the complete care package?

A) 59400
B) 59409, 59410
C) 59409, 59400
D) 59410

8. A patient undergoes a needle biopsy of the prostate, and during the same session, an excisional biopsy is performed on a different prostate lesion. Which coding scenario is correct?

A) 55700, 55706-51
B) 55700, 55705-51
C) 55706
D) 55700, 55705

9. A patient undergoes an IVF procedure that includes oocyte retrieval and embryo transfer via intrauterine method. How should these procedures be coded?

A) 58970, 58974
B) 58976, 58673-51
C) 58974-51, 58976
D) 58970, 58976-51

10. A laparoscopic nephrolithotomy is performed to remove a kidney stone. The procedure also involves the use of lithotripsy to break down larger fragments. How should these procedures be coded?

A) 50060, 50590-51
B) 50561, 50590-51
C) 50590, 50075
D) 50561

KEY ANSWERS

1. **C) 50220, 52332-51**

   Explanation: The total nephrectomy via an open approach is coded as 50220. The ureteral stent insertion during cystoscopy should be coded separately as 52332. Modifier 51 is applied because multiple procedures were performed in the same session.

2. **D) 50543, 50590-51**

   Explanation: The laparoscopic partial nephrectomy is coded as 50543, and the percutaneous lithotripsy as 50590. Modifier 51 is used for multiple procedures performed on the same site during the same session.

3. **D) 52355**

   Explanation: According to the guidelines, when both biopsy and excision are performed on the same lesion, only the excision (52355) is coded, as the biopsy is considered part of the excision procedure.

4. **B) 58552**

   Explanation: CPT 58552 is for a laparoscopic-assisted vaginal hysterectomy (LAVH) with bilateral salpingo-oophorectomy. It's important to verify that the procedure involves both the uterus and the ovaries/tubes, which differentiates it from the other options.

5. **B) 52320, 52332-51**

   Explanation: 52320 is for the therapeutic cystourethroscopy with lithotripsy, and **52332-51** is for the stent insertion, with the modifier **-51** for multiple procedures.

6. **A) 56630**

    Explanation: 56630 is the CPT code for a partial vulvectomy involving less than 80% of the vulva, including superficial and deep subcutaneous tissue.

7. **A) 59400**

    Explanation 59400 is the code that includes vaginal delivery with episiotomy, forceps, and comprehensive antepartum and postpartum care.

8. **D) 55700, 55705**

    Explanation 55700 is for a needle biopsy of the prostate, and **55705** is for an excisional biopsy, performed on a different lesion during the same session.

9. **D) 58970, 58976-51**

    Explanation 58970 is for oocyte retrieval, and **58976-51** is for embryo transfer via intrauterine method, with the modifier **-51** for multiple procedures.

10. **D) 50561**

    Explanation 50561 is the correct code for a laparoscopic nephrolithotomy, which includes the removal of kidney stones and the use of lithotripsy during the procedure.

Chapter 8

Nervous System - Coding Guidelines (60000)

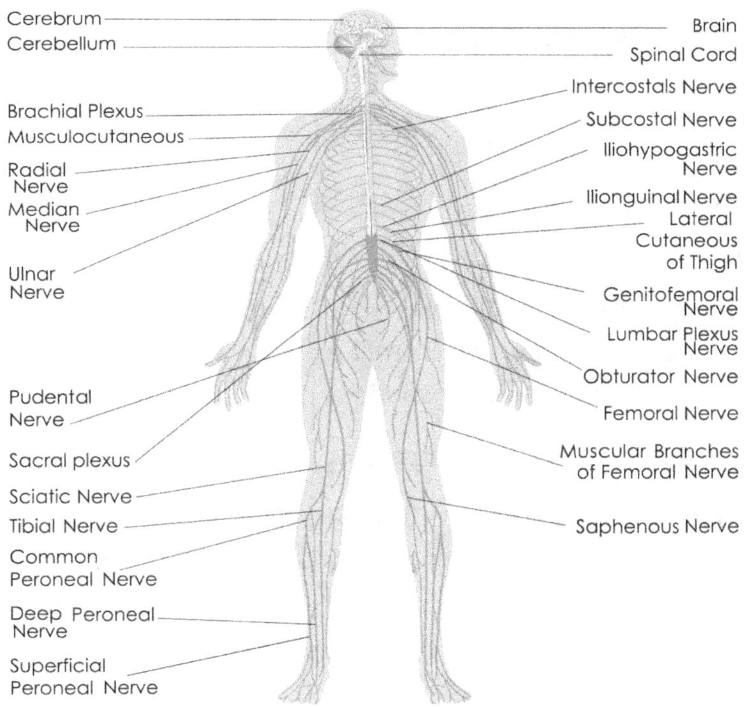

There are 31 pairs of nerves

o   8 – Cervical

o   12 – Thoracic

- o   5 – Lumbar
- o   5 – Sacral
- o   1 – Coccygeal

Spine bones

- o   7 – Cervical
- o   12 Thoracic
- o   5 – Lumbar
- o   1 – Sacral (5 bones fused)

Organs of Nervous System

- o   Brain
- o   Spinal Cord
- o   Nerves

Thyroidectomy

It is surgical removal of all or part of the thyroid gland, which is located in the front of the neck. The thyroid gland releases thyroid hormone, which controls many critical functions of the body.

Coding Guidelines for Thyroidectomy

Thyroidectomy ranges from 60100 – 60281 and includes Lobectomy, Partial Lobectomy, Bi-Lobectomy. Code according to the procedure mentioned.

Burr Hole

Burr holes are small holes that a neurosurgeon makes in the skull. Burr holes are used to help relieve pressure on the brain when fluid, such as blood, builds up and starts to compress brain tissue.

Coding Guidelines For Burr Hole

1. Check for the appropriate procedure and thereby the codes:

i.   Ventricular puncture

ii. Implantation of catheter/monitoring device

iii. Hematoma release

2. If burr hole is accompanied with craniotomy / craniectomy, do not code for burr hole, only code for craniotomy or craniectomy.

Skull Base Surgery (Coding Guidelines)

Check the following before coding:

i.   Approach – (Anterior, middle or posterior)

ii. Definitive (Anterior, middle or posterior)

iii. Repair

iv. Do not use modifier 62 for skull-based surgery

v.   Use modifier 51 if the surgeon has performed multiple procedure during the surgery.

Cerebral Spinal Fluid (CSF) Shunt

Placement of cerebral spinal fluid (CSF) shunt systems to treat hydrocephalus is a common medical procedure and a life-saving treatment for many patients. These shunt systems drain excess fluid from the brain to another part of the body where the fluid is absorbed as part of the circulatory process.

Coding Guidelines

i.   Insertion or placement

ii. Removal

iii. Replacement of CSF shunt system

iv. Replacement of valves (proximal or ventricular vs distal vs obstructed valve)

Spinal Cord (Coding Guidelines)

i. Spinal procedure – Which spinal procedure is done (laminectomy, discectomy, vertebral, corpectomy etc.)

ii. Epidural injection code ranges from 64479 – 64484

iii. Paravertebral / facet injection ranges from 64490 – 64484

Eyes – Coding Guidelines

Strabismus Surgery – Eye muscle surgery, treats misaligned eyes that haven't responded to other treatments.

In case of Retinal **Detachment Repair**, check the procedure, if it is scleral buckling, cryotherapy, laser or photocoagulation. Choose codes ranging from 67101, 67105, 67107, 67113, 67141, 67145.

i. **Retinal Detachment:** It happens when retina is pulled away from its normal position at the back of one's eye.

ii. **Scleral Buckling:** is a type of eye surgery to correct a detached retina and restore vision.

iii. **Cryotherapy:** It consists of the transmission of freezing temperatures to the retina, by applying a very cold probe to the outside of the eye.

iv. **Photocoagulation:** Laser photocoagulation is eye surgery utilizing heat from a laser to shrink or destroy abnormal blood vessels in the retina.

Intraocular Lens – Coding Guidelines

i. Extracapsular v/s intracapsular

ii. Extracapsular – 66982, 66984

iii. Intracapsular – 66983

iv. Placement of secondary lens without cataract removal – 66985

v. Exchange – 66986

Ear Codes

i. Removal of foreign body from external auditory canal (without general anaesthesia): 69200

ii. Removal of foreign body from external auditory canal (with general anaesthesia): 69205

iii. Removal impacted cerumen using irrigation/lavage (unilateral): 69209

iv. Removal impacted cerumen requiring instrumentation (unilateral): 69210

v. Mastoidectomy (complete): 69502

vi. Mastoidectomy (modified radical): 69505

vii. Mastoidectomy (radical): 69511

QUIZ

1. A patient undergoes a complete thyroidectomy followed by a partial lobectomy on the contralateral lobe during the same surgical session. Which codes and modifiers should be reported?

   A) 60240, 60220-51
   B) 60240, 60220-59
   C) 60252, 60240-51
   D) 60240, 60252-51

2. A patient with hydrocephalus undergoes the insertion of a CSF shunt system. The surgeon also replaces the obstructed valve in the existing shunt. How should these procedures be coded?

   A) 62223, 62230-51
   B) 62225, 62230
   C) 62223, 62258-51
   D) 62258, 62230

3. During a skull base surgery, the surgeon performs an anterior cranial fossa approach, followed by definitive tumor removal and reconstruction. What coding considerations should be applied?

   A) Modifier 62 should be used for the approach.
   B) Modifier 51 should be used for multiple procedures.
   C) Only code the definitive procedure without any modifiers.
   D) Code each stage separately with modifier 62.

4. A patient undergoes a burr hole procedure for the release of a subdural hematoma, followed by craniotomy for further exploration. How should these procedures be coded?

   A) Code both the burr hole and craniotomy.
   B) Only code for the craniotomy.
   C) Use a modifier 59 for the burr hole.
   D) Code the burr hole with modifier 51.

5. A surgeon performs a laminectomy at the L4-L5 level with an epidural injection. Which codes and modifiers should be used for accurate coding?

    A) 63030, 64483-51
    B) 63047, 64479-59
    C) 63047, 64483-51
    D) 63030, 64479-59

6. A patient requires removal of a foreign body from the external auditory canal under general anesthesia, and during the same session, a modified radical mastoidectomy is performed. What is the appropriate coding?

    A) 69205, 69505-51
    B) 69200, 69511-51
    C) 69205, 69511-51
    D) 69205, 69505-59

7. A patient undergoes scleral buckling for retinal detachment repair and later requires laser photocoagulation in the same session. Which codes should be reported?

    A) 67107, 67141-51
    B) 67107, 67145-51
    C) 67113, 67145-51
    D) 67108, 67113-51

8. A patient undergoes extracapsular cataract extraction with the placement of an intraocular lens, followed by a secondary lens placement without cataract removal. What coding should be used?

    A) 66982, 66985
    B) 66984, 66985
    C) 66983, 66986
    D) 66984, 66986

9. A neurosurgeon performs a ventricular puncture using a burr hole technique. During the same session, a catheter is implanted for CSF monitoring. Which coding combination is accurate?

    A) 61107, 62225-51
    B) 61154, 62230-51
    C) 61154, 62225-51
    D) 61107, 62230-51

10. A patient presents with a detached retina and requires cryotherapy followed by scleral buckling in the same session. How should the procedures be coded?

    A) 67113, 67101-51
    B) 67101, 67107-51
    C) 67113, 67108-51
    D) 67108, 67141-51

KEY ANSWERS

1. **A) 60240, 60220-51**

   Explanation: 60240 is the CPT code for a complete thyroidectomy, and **60220** is for a partial lobectomy. The modifier **-51** is used because both procedures were performed in the same session.

2. **C) 62223, 62258-51**

   Explanation: 62223 codes for the insertion of a CSF shunt, while **62258** codes for the replacement of the obstructed valve, with the **-51** modifier indicating multiple procedures.

3. **B) Modifier 51 should be used for multiple procedures.**

   Explanation: Modifier **-51** is appropriate when multiple procedures are performed during skull base surgery. Modifier **-62** is not used in skull base surgery coding.

4. **B) Only code for the craniotomy.**

   Explanation: If a burr hole is followed by a craniotomy or craniectomy, only the craniotomy/craniectomy should be coded, per the guidelines.

5. **C) 63047, 64483-51**

   Explanation: 63047 is for the laminectomy, and **64483** is for the epidural injection at the lumbar region, with the **-51** modifier indicating multiple procedures.

6. **C) 69205, 69511-5**

   Explanation: 69205 is for the removal of a foreign body under general anesthesia, and **69511** is for a modified radical mastoidectomy, with the **-51** modifier indicating multiple procedures.

7. **B) 67107, 67145-51**

   Explanation: 67107 codes for scleral buckling, and **67145** codes for laser photocoagulation, with the **-51** modifier indicating multiple procedures.

8. **B) 66984, 66985**

   Explanation: 66984 codes for extracapsular cataract extraction with intraocular lens placement, and **66985** codes for secondary lens placement without cataract removal.

9. **C) 61154, 62225-51**

   Explanation: 61154 codes for a ventricular puncture using a burr hole, and **62225** codes for the implantation of a catheter, with **-51** indicating multiple procedures.

10. **B) 67101, 67107-51**

    Explanation: 67101 codes for cryotherapy for retinal detachment, and **67107** is for scleral buckling, with **-51** indicating multiple procedures performed during the same session.

Chapter 9

Radiology – Coding Guidelines (70000)

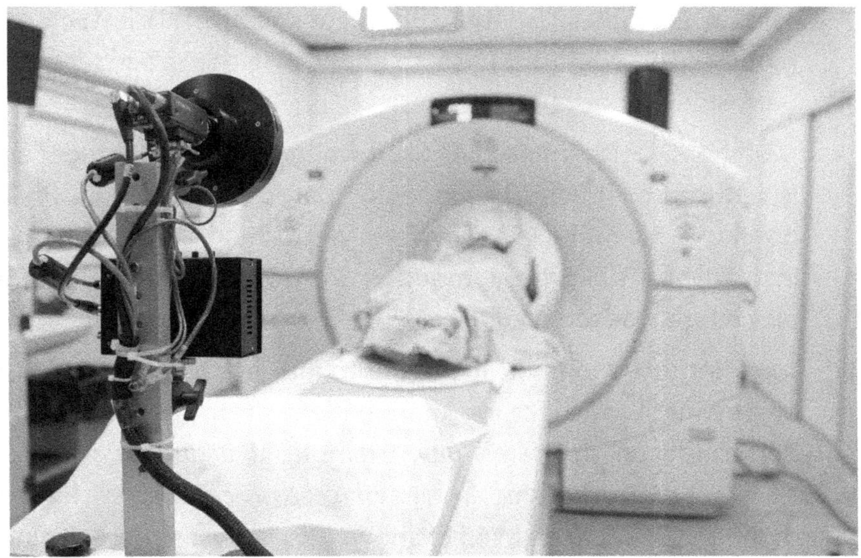

Important Modifiers

i. Modifier 26 - Modifier 26 indicates that only the professional component of a service or procedure is being billed. Example: A physician interpreting a radiology report but not performing the imaging study would use this modifier to indicate they are billing only for the interpretation.

ii. Modifier TC - Modifier TC refers to the technical component of a service or procedure. Example: A radiology facility performing an MRI would use this modifier to indicate they are billing only for the technical aspects of the procedure.

iii. Modifier LT & RT - LT (Left Side): Used to specify that a procedure was performed on the left side of the body. RT (Right Side): Used to specify that a procedure was performed on the right side of the body. Example: If a patient had an injection in the left knee, you would use modifier LT. If the injection was in the right knee, you would use modifier RT.

iv. Modifier 50 - Modifier 50 is used to indicate that a procedure was performed on both sides of the body during the same session. Example: If a patient undergoes a bilateral mastectomy, modifier 50 would be used to show that the procedure was performed on both breasts.

v. Modifier 52 - Modifier 52 is used when a service or procedure is reduced or limited in scope compared to what is normally provided. Example: If a physician performed a partial biopsy instead of a full biopsy, modifier 52 would indicate that the procedure was reduced.

vi. Modifier 59 - Modifier 59 is used to indicate that a procedure or service is distinct or independent from other services performed on the same day. Example: If a patient received an injection in the arm and a separate procedure on the leg, modifier 59 would be used to show these services were distinct and not bundled together.

vii. Modifier 76 - Modifier 76 indicates that a procedure or service was repeated by the same physician or provider. Example: If a patient required a repeat echocardiogram on the same day, modifier 76 would be used to show the procedure was repeated.

viii. Modifier 77 - Modifier 77 is used when a procedure or service is repeated by a different physician or provider. Example: If a different physician performs a repeat test or procedure on the same day, modifier 77 would be used to show the service was repeated by another physician.

Body Plane

i. Sagittal plane – Divide body into right and left side.

ii. Transverse / Horizontal Plane – Divide the body into top and bottom half.

iii. Frontal / Coronal – Divide the body into front and back section.

Projection

i. Anterior to Posterior – From front to back.

ii. Lateral – Left to right side.

iii. Posterior – anterior – Back to front.

iv. Oblique – At an angle.

v. Cone – Focused or spot view.

X Ray – Coding Guideline

i. If a single view of wrist x-ray is performed then append modifier 52 (Reduced service) with CPT 73100 (Because of CPT code description states it's 2 views).

ii. If four or more views of wrist x- rays are taken no need to append any modifier with CPT 73110 since the CPT description is stating that it's minimum of 3 views.

iii. If bilateral wrist x- rays are taken then we can code either using modifier 50 (Bilateral procedures modifier) or modifier RT & LT.

iv. We will code for maximum views, in case it is specifically mentioned. However, if nothing is mentioned code for at least one view.

Computed Tomography (CT) Scan – Coding Guidelines

It is a non-invasive imaging technology that produces three dimensional detailed anatomical images. It is often used for disease detection, diagnosis, and treatment monitoring. CT scan codes are arranged based on contrast material used or not.

First Standalone code would be **without contrast** study and followed by two intended codes (Second code is for with contrast and the third code would be with and without contrast study).

Types of Radiation Treatment Delivery

Which type of radiation is given?

i. X-ray (photon), including conventional and intensity modulated radiation therapy (IMRT) beams:

ii. Electron beams

iii. Neutron beams

iv. Proton beams

Radiation Treatment Management (RTM) – 77427 – 77499

It is reported in units of five fractions or treatment sessions, regardless of the actual time in which the services are finished. The doctor will not give all radiation therapy at one go. The radiations are usually given in a **block of five.**

77427 – Radiation treatment management, 5 treatments.

If the treatment is given for 3 months, multiply with 77427. If after giving radiation therapy for 3 months, only one or two treatments are required, it will be free and there will be zero charge. Similarly if the patient receives four treatments instead of five, then also 77427 code will be used. The patient will be charged for full five treatments.

77431 – Radiation therapy management with complete course of therapy consisting of one or two fractions only.

Radiation Treatment Delivery V/S Radiation Treatment Management

Radiation treatment deliver is different from radiation treatment management. In radiation treatment delivery MEV each session is reported separately based on complexity. Radiation treatment delivery takes into account the type of radiation used.

Radiation treatment management, radiation therapy is given in units of five.

QUIZ

1. A radiologist interprets a CT scan of the chest with and without contrast, but the imaging was performed by a different facility. Which coding and modifier combination is correct?

   A) 71260
   B) 71270-26
   C) 71275-TC
   D) 71270-26, 71275-TC

2. During a diagnostic session, a patient undergoes X-rays of both wrists, with four views taken for each wrist. What is the correct coding and modifier usage?

   A) 73100, 73110-50
   B) 73110-RT, 73110-LT
   C) 73100-52, 73100-50
   D) 73110-50

3. A radiation oncologist manages a patient's treatment over four weeks, providing a total of 20 radiation therapy sessions. Which code accurately reflects the management of these sessions?

   A) 77427 x 4
   B) 77427 x 5
   C) 77431
   D) 77499

4. A patient receives a photon beam radiation treatment daily for 10 days. The complexity of the treatment was high. What is the correct way to code this?

   A) 77427 x 2
   B) 77427 x 1, 77431
   C) 77431 x 2
   D) 77412 x 10

5. A repeat chest X-ray is performed by the same provider later on the same day to check the resolution of a pneumothorax. Which coding and modifier combination is correct?

    A) 71020, 71020-77
    B) 71020-59, 71020
    C) 71020-26, 71020-TC
    D) 71020, 71020-76

6. A patient undergoes an MRI of the brain performed by a radiology facility, with the radiologist only providing the interpretation and report. How should this be coded?

    A) 70551-26
    B) 70552-TC
    C) 70551-TC, 70552-26
    D) 70553-26

7. A patient receives an injection in the left shoulder and undergoes a separate procedure on the right knee on the same day. Which modifier should be used to indicate the procedures are distinct?

    A) 50
    B) 52
    C) 59
    D) LT, RT

8. During an imaging session, an X-ray of the pelvis was performed with anterior-posterior and oblique views. Which projection term best describes the oblique view?

    A) Anterior-posterior
    B) Posterior-anterior
    C) Sagittal
    D) At an angle

9. A diagnostic radiology service is provided with both the professional and technical components by the same provider. Which modifier, if any, should be appended?

   A) 26
   B) TC
   C) 59
   D) None

10. A patient receives radiation therapy management consisting of one fraction due to the patient's limited tolerance. How should this be coded?

   A) 77427
   B) 77431
   C) 77499
   D) 77427-52

KEY ANSWERS

1. **B) 71270-26**

   Explanation: 71270 is the CPT code for a CT scan of the chest with and without contrast. The **-26** modifier is used to indicate that only the professional component (interpretation) of the service was performed by the radiologist.

2. **D) 73110-50**

   Explanation: 73110 is the CPT code for wrist X-rays with three or more views. The **-50** modifier indicates that the procedure was performed bilaterally.

3. **A) 77427 x 4**

   Explanation: 77427 is used for radiation treatment management of five sessions. Since the patient had 20 sessions over four weeks, **77427** should be reported four times.

4. **A) 77427 x 2**

   Explanation: 77427 represents radiation treatment management for five sessions. For 10 sessions, **77427** would be reported twice. The complexity is factored into the delivery codes, not the management codes.

5. **D) 71020, 71020-76**

   Explanation: 71020 is the CPT code for a chest X-ray, two views. Modifier -76 indicates that the procedure was repeated by the same provider on the same day.

6. **A) 70551-26**

   Explanation: 70551 is the CPT code for an MRI of the brain without contrast. The -26 modifier indicates that only the professional component (interpretation) is being billed.

7. **C) 59**

   Explanation: Modifier -**59** is used to indicate that procedures performed on the same day are distinct and should not be bundled together.

8. **D) At an angle**

   Explanation: The **oblique** projection refers to an imaging view taken at an angle.

9. **D) None**

   Explanation: When both the professional and technical components are provided by the same provider, no modifier is necessary as the full service is being billed.

10. **B) 77431**

    Explanation: 77431 is used for radiation therapy management where the complete course consists of only one or two fractions.

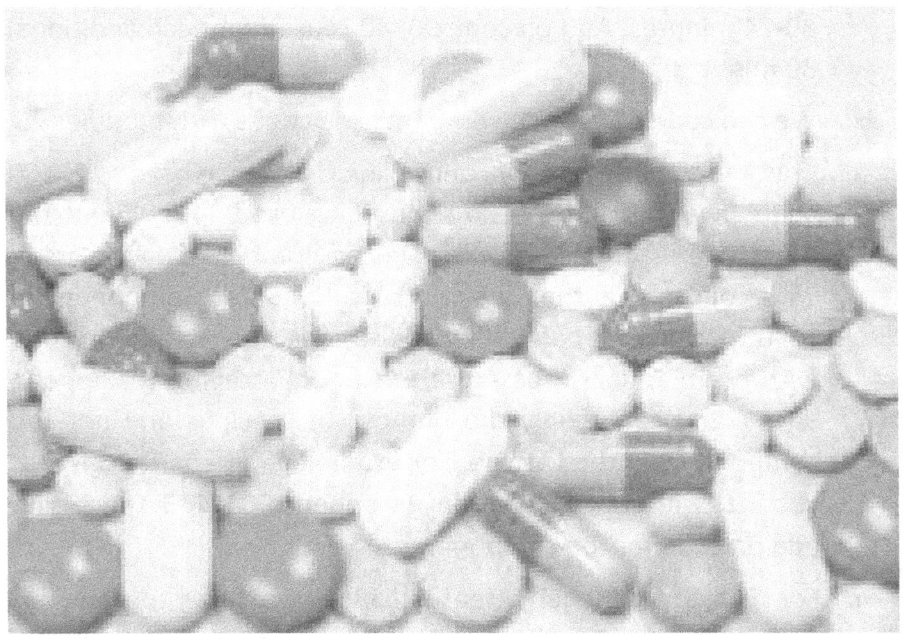

i. Before coding check if the injection is given by the doctor or by a nurse.

ii. Injections are coded by routes. In case it is given intramuscularly, report 96372.

iii. **Injection, catheterization, angiography and supervision and interpretation are all bundled in 93458**

iv. Hydration therapy is 96360, you will append 96361 if hydration is given for more than **30 minutes.**

v. The subcategory guidelines for the audiologic function test with medical diagnostic evaluation state to add modifier 52, if only one ear is checked by the doctor. Modifier 52 is used for reduced procedure.

vi. Administration of vaccines are reported according to the route and the age of the patient.

vii. **Never use Modifier 51 in entire chapter of Medicine.**

viii. Psychotherapy for crisis is reported with code 90839 for the first 30-74 minutes. Add on code 90840 is used for each additional 30 minutes.

ix. We can code E&M code with medicine codes with modifier 25

x. Check for counselling – if counselling is done we have to 90460 code always. If there is no counselling use 90471. Count the number of vaccines, for example the number of vaccine is 4, with counselling, then we will code 90460*4. Component of each vaccine is appended by 90461 code, it is an add-on code with no modifier. In case there is no counselling we append 90471 and count only the number of vaccines and not the components in the vaccine. For example if a patient is given 3 vaccines without consultation, we append 90471*3, there is no add on code for the components.

xi. For End Stage Renal Disease (ESRD), we have to code for outpatient. Keep a watch on the key terms, full month, complete assessment, monthly service, then we have to code the codes (90951-90966) based on the age of the patients and face to face visits.

xii. Psychotherapy topic check the time given in scenario.

QUIZ

1. A 45-year-old patient receives an intramuscular injection administered by a nurse, followed by a 90-minute hydration therapy. How should these services be coded?

   A) 96372, 96360 x 2
   B) 96372, 96360, 96361 x 2
   C) 96372, 96361 x 2
   D) 96372, 96360, 96361

2. During a routine visit, a patient receives three vaccines without any counselling. How should this be coded?

   A) 90460 x 3
   B) 90471, 90471-51 x 2
   C) 90471 x 3
   D) 90460, 90461 x 2

3. A physician performs a catheterization, angiography, and provides supervision and interpretation during a coronary angiogram. Which code should be reported?

   A) 93458
   B) 93556, 93566
   C) 93460, 93555-52
   D) 93458, 93555

4. A 60-year-old patient undergoing End Stage Renal Disease (ESRD) treatment has two face-to-face visits in a month. What code should be used to report the monthly service?

   A) 90957
   B) 90960
   C) 90961
   D) 90958

5. A physician spends 90 minutes with a patient in crisis, providing psychotherapy. How should this be coded?

    A) 90839, 90840 x 2
    B) 90839, 90840
    C) 90832, 90834-52
    D) 90837

6. A paediatric patient receives two vaccines, one with counselling and one without. How should the administration be coded?

    A) 90460 x 2
    B) 90460, 90471
    C) 90471 x 2
    D) 90460, 90461

7. A patient receives an intramuscular injection from a physician during an evaluation and management (E/M) visit, with the visit focused on discussing the patient's ongoing condition. How should the injection and E/M service be coded?

    A) 96372, 99213-25
    B) 96372, 99213
    C) 96372, 99213-59
    D) 96372-52, 99213-25

KEY ANSWER

1. **B) 96372, 96360, 96361 (96361 once only)**

   Explanation: 96372 is used for the intramuscular injection. **96360** is used for the first hour of hydration therapy, and **96361** is added for each additional 30 minutes. Since the hydration lasted 90 minutes, **96361** is reported twice.

2. **C) 90471 x 3**

   Explanation: 90471 is used for the administration of vaccines without counselling. The number of vaccines administered (3) is counted, and **90471** is reported for each vaccine. Since no counselling was provided, there is no need for **90460** or **90461**.

3. **A) 93458**

   Explanation: 93458 is a comprehensive code that bundles catheterization, angiography, and the supervision and interpretation components. No additional codes are needed as they are included in **93458**.

4. **B) 90960**

   Explanation: 90960 is used for ESRD services, covering a full month of care for a patient aged 20 years or older who has received two to three face-to-face visits.

5. **B) 90839, 90840**

   Explanation: 90839 is used for the first 30-74 minutes of psychotherapy for a crisis. Since the session lasted 90 minutes, **90840** (an add-on code for each additional 30 minutes) is also reported once.

6. **B) 90460, 90471**

   Explanation: 90460 is used for the vaccine with counselling. **90471** is used for the vaccine administered without counselling. Since only two vaccines are given, **90461** (which is used for additional components of the same vaccine) is not needed.

7. **A) 96372, 99213-25**

   Explanation: 96372 is used for the intramuscular injection. **99213** is used for the E/M service. Since the E/M service is separately identifiable, **modifier -25** is added to indicate that it is distinct from the injection procedure.

Evaluation & Management – Coding Guidelines (99000)

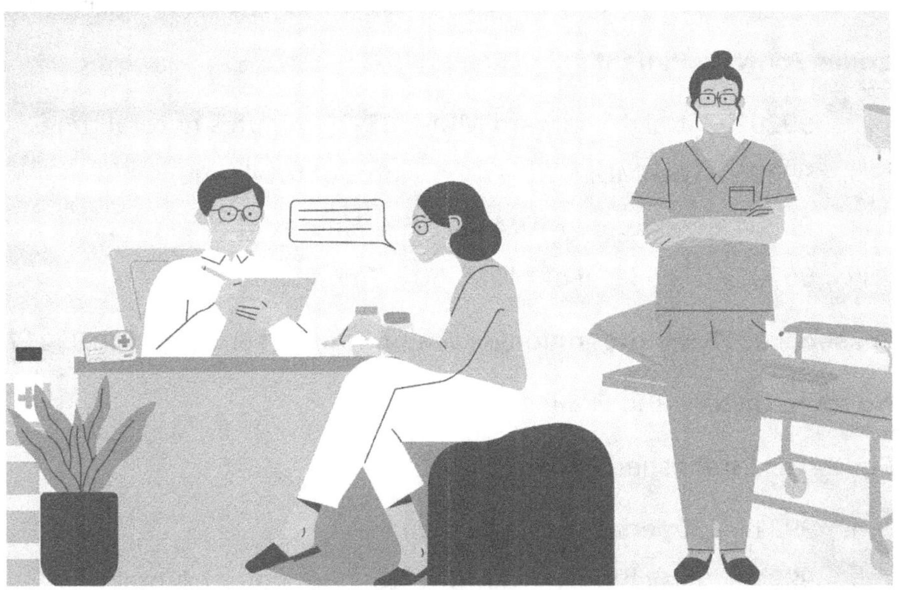

New Patient

A new patient is one who has received any professional services from the physician or other qualified health care professional or another physician or other qualified health care professional of the **exact same specialty** and **subspecialty** who belongs to the same group practice. New patient requires extensive documentation.

Established Patient

An established patient is one who has received professional services from the physician or other qualified health care professional or another physician or other qualified health care professional of the **exact same specialty and subspecialty** who belongs to the same group practice, **within the past three years.**

Office or Other Outpatient Service

Office visit codes are subcategorized as new or established patient. The codes are selected based on time and Medical Decision Making (MDM).

Codes For New Patient

   i.   99202 – Straight forward MDM. 15-29 minutes of total time.

   ii.   99203 – Low MDM. 30 – 44 minutes of total time.

   iii.   99204 – Moderate MDM. 45 – 59 minutes of total time.

   iv.   99205 – High level of MDM. 60 – 74 minutes

For services 75 minutes or longer use prolonged services code 99417

No more History and Exam

Codes For Established Patient

   i.   99211 – Supervised clinical team.

   ii.   99212 - Straight forward MDM. 10-19 minutes of total time.

   iii.   99213 - Low MDM. 20 – 29 minutes of total time.

   iv.   99214 - Moderate MDM. 30 – 39 minutes of total time.

   v.   99215 - High level of MDM. 40 – 45 minutes

For services 55 minutes or longer use prolonged services code 99417

99211 – This code from established patient, is outpatient office code. This particular code is not coded based on time and MDM. It is called a nursing staff or a clinical staff code. Even the physician's service is not used and a nurse's service for the patient is used, we may use this particular code.

Hospital Observation Services

Let us discuss the difference between observation services and inpatient.

i. Observation services are used when the patient is kept just for observation and the physician is not actively treating the patient.

ii. While inpatient service is when the patient is hospitalized for some ailment and the doctor is actively treating him.

iii. If a doctor from some specialty sees the patient for the first time, then initial service code is coded.

iv. During same hospitalization another doctor from different specialty or subspecialty visits the patient then initial service code is coded.

v. If the patient is in observation status and the patient's health condition deteriorates and the patient is admitted in the hospital, initial service code is coded.

Codes For Initial Hospital Care

i. 99221 – Straight forward / Low MDM 40 minutes

ii. 99222 – Moderate MDM – 55 minutes

iii. 99223 – High MDM 75 minutes

Hospital Inpatient or Observation Care Services (Including Admission & Discharge)

Number of Hours	Discharged Calendar Date	Report Codes
< 8 hours	Same calendar date as initial hospital inpatient or observation care service.	99221 99222 99223

8 or more hours	Same calendar date as initial hospital inpatient or observation care service.	99234 99235 99236
< 8 hours	Different calendar date as initial hospital inpatient or observation care service	99221 99222 99223
8 or more hours	Different calendar date as initial hospital inpatient or observation care service	99221 99222 99223 and 99238,99239

We code as initial hospital service if the patient is admitted and discharged on the same day and hospitalization was less than 8 hours. Discharge codes are not coded, only initial service codes ranging from 99221 – 99223 are coded.

When the patient is hospitalized and discharged on the same day, however, hospitalization is more than 8 hours, we use 99234-99236. These codes are used for the same calendar day.

If the patient is hospitalized for 6 hours. He is admitted at 9 pm on day one and discharged at 3 am on day two. Even when the calendar date has changed still the number of hours the patient is hospitalized for is less than 8 and hence we will use the inpatient hospitalization code from 99221-99223.

99238-99239 codes are admission and **discharge codes** based on time and not on MDM. The patient must be hospitalized for greater than 8 hours and the discharge date is different calendar dates.

Subsequent Hospital Inpatient or Observation Care

    i. When the patient receives subsequent service from a physician or other physician of the same specialty, then it is coded as a subsequent care.

ii. If the same physician who treated the patient on day one, meets the patient on day two, three and seventh respectively, the code will be subsequent care code.

iii. Codes are chosen on time and MDM

Codes For Subsequent Care

i. 99231 – Straight forward / Low MDM 25 minutes

ii. 99232 – Moderate MDM – 35 minutes

iii. 99233 – High MDM 50 minutes

Consultation

For any kind of consultation 3 R criteria must be met.

i. R- Reference

ii. R- Review

iii. R – Reporting back

Check if the consultation is done in office or hospital, based on that codes must be chosen. Consultation codes are based on time and MDM.

Emergency Department – An emergency department is defined as an organized hospital-based facility for the provision of unscheduled episodic services to patients who present for immediate medical attention.

These codes have no subcategories. These codes do not have time as the deciding factor, only MDM.

Whenever you choose a code you do not give preference to the place of service example emergency department. You focus on type of service which is emergency.

Critical Care Service

A critical illness or injury acutely injures one or more vital organ systems, such that there is high probability of imminent or life threatening deterioration in the patient's condition. Critical organs are brain, heart, lung, kidney.

Critical care codes are based on time and not on MDM.

Total Duration of Critical Care Codes	
Less Than 30 minutes	Appropriate E/M codes
30 - 74	99291*1
75-104 minutes	99291*1 AND 99292 * 1
105 - 134 minutes	99291 * 1 AND 99292 * 2
135 - 164 minutes	99291 * 1 AND 99292 *3
165 - 194 minutes	99291 * 1 AND 99292 * 4
195 minutes or longer	99291 AND 99292 as appropriate

If the consultation is less than 30 minutes, critical care codes will not be used. Inpatient codes will be used instead.

99291 is the critical care code and 99292 is an add on code. These two codes can be used for inpatient and outpatient for "Adults". However, **for inpatient neonates** there are different critical care codes. Be careful.

Nursing Facility Discharge Services

When a patient is getting discharged from nursing facility 99315-99316 codes are used. But the discharge must be on different calendar dates. If it is the same date then initial nursing facility codes are used.

Standby Service

99360 Standby service, requiring prolonged attendance, each 30 minutes. The standby physician will not do anything, the physician will just be with the patient. For example, during complicated child birth, a paediatrician simply stands and observes the delivery process. If only needed the paediatrician will get involved. Even if the physician is a standby, he/she will be paid for the time. The standby physician must complete 30 minutes, if it is 29 minutes, the service provided won't be coded.

Medical Team Conference

99366 – 99368 – Minimum 3 doctors from different specialties have seen and treated the patient within past 60 days. These are time based codes.

99366 – With direct patient contact.

99367-99368 – Without patient direct contact. The patient need not be there in person, the physicians may discuss and create plans.

Care Plan Oversight Service

One physician is taking care of all the complaints of a patient. One individual is overseeing the patient's condition (For example, a GP). He is supervising and liaising the patient with other specialist doctors.

99374-99375 – Supervision of home health, time specific code.

99377-99378 – Supervision of hospice care, time specific code.

99379-99380 – Supervision of nursing facility, time specific code.

Preventive Medicine Services

Preventive medicine codes are categorized into three parts:

i. When the patient is healthy but he needs advice to increase stamina or how to lead a healthy life. **99381-99387 – New Patient. 99391 – 99397 – Established Patient**

ii. People with a possibility of disease, they are healthy but have a family history of for example pulmonary disease or Type II Diabetes. Out of concern they approach the physician. **99401-99404**

iii. People who are exposing themselves to risk, smokers, drug addicts etc. They may approach the doctor for help to lead a normal life. **99406 – 99407 – Tobacco use. 99408-99409 – Other substance use**

Preventive Medicine Group Counselling

When the physician does group counselling for a set of people. These codes are based on time. Codes are 99411 – 99412

Non-Face-to Face Service

Telephone Services – For example, during Covid times, telephone services were used. Codes can be used once the doctor has seen the patient earlier. The doctor must have seen the doctor in the past 7 days. These codes are time-based codes. Telephone codes cannot be coded with face to face consultation. Codes are from the range 99441-99443.

Online Digital Evaluation and Management Services – When the doctor consults the patient through hospital apps or emails. Guidelines are same as telephone consultation.

Interprofessional Telephone / Internet / Electronic Health Record Consultation

The patient's health condition is stored electronically. This data is available across hospital and clinics across the US. These are time-based codes, how much time the doctor spends consulting over the data or how much time the doctor takes going through the data. Codes range from 99447-99452

Newborn Care Services

Whenever the child is born either in the hospital or is born outside and taken to the hospital immediately.

99460 – Initial care when the child is born in a hospital.

99461 – When the child is born outside the hospital and brought into the hospital immediately.

99462 – Subsequent hospital care.

99463 – When the neonate is admitted and discharged on the same date.

Delivery / Birthing Room Attendance & Resuscitation Services

Codes range from 99464 – 99465. 99464 - When the doctor is required to stabilize the child's health condition.

99465 – The doctor resuscitates the child, if the child is not breathing and the doctor helps the child breathe. If the doctor is not doing anything, use the standby code.

Paediatric Critical Care Patient Transport

99466 – Terminally ill neonate is transported from one facility to another. During transport, physician gives face to face service.

+99467 – Each additional 30 minutes.

99485 – 99486 – Transport but non-face-face service provided but during transportation the physician is going to speak to transport team.

99468 – Initial critical care neonate 28 days or younger, per day service.

99469 – Subsequent, whenever the critical care treatment is given to the neonate the same day by the same physician or the subsequent day by same or another physician.

Initial & Continuing Intensive Care Services

Intensive care is different from critical care. If a neonate or paediatric is critically ill, intensive monitoring must be done. Then intensive care codes are used.

QUIZ

1. A patient is hospitalized and receives subsequent care from the same physician on days two and three. The MDM on day two is straightforward, while on day three, the MDM is moderate. How should these subsequent care services be coded?

   A) 99231 on both days
   B) 99231 on day two, 99232 on day three
   C) 99232 on both days
   D) 99233 on day three, 99231 on day two

2. A patient is admitted to the hospital for observation and discharged on the same day after 9 hours. How should the physician's services be coded?

   A) 99234
   B) 99221
   C) 99235
   D) 99222

3. A newborn is delivered in a hospital and requires stabilization by a physician immediately after birth. Which code should be reported for the physician's service?

   A) 99464
   B) 99465
   C) 99460
   D) 99462

4. A 55-year-old patient with a history of Type II diabetes consults a physician for preventive care to manage potential complications due to his family history of cardiovascular disease. How should this be coded?

   A) 99401
   B) 99397

C) 99387
D) 99403

5. A physician provides 40 minutes of critical care to a 65-year-old patient with acute respiratory failure in an outpatient setting. How should the services be coded?

    A) 99291
    B) 99291, 99292
    C) 99215
    D) 99466

6. A pediatrician is on standby during a high-risk delivery but does not actively intervene. The physician was present for 45 minutes. How should this service be coded?

    A) 99464
    B) 99360
    C) 99465
    D) 99460

7. A patient is seen in an outpatient office by a new physician for 50 minutes. The physician documents a moderate level of Medical Decision Making (MDM). Which code should be used?

    A) 99203
    B) 99204
    C) 99205
    D) 99417

8. A physician supervises a clinical team providing care to an established patient in an outpatient setting. No MDM or time documentation is provided. How should this service be coded?

    A) 99212
    B) 99213
    C) 99211
    D) 99441

9. A physician provides 15 minutes of consultation over the phone to a patient they have seen within the last 7 days. How should this service be coded?

   A) 99441
   B) 99443
   C) 99211
   D) 99421

10. A critically ill neonate is transferred to a different facility, and the attending physician provides face-to-face care during the transport. The transport took 50 minutes. How should the service be coded?

   A) 99466, 99467
   B) 99468
   C) 99466
   D) 99485

KEY ANSWER

1. **B) 99231 on day two, 99232 on day three**

   Explanation: 99231 is used for subsequent care with straightforward or low MDM, while **99232** is used for subsequent care with moderate MDM. Since day two involves straightforward MDM and day three involves moderate MDM, **99231** and **99232** are the appropriate codes.

2. **C) 99235**

   Explanation: When a patient is admitted for observation and discharged on the same day after more than 8 hours, the appropriate code is chosen from **99234-99236** based on the MDM. **99235** is used for moderate MDM.

3. **A) 99464**

   Explanation: 99464 is used when a physician is required to stabilize the newborn's condition immediately after birth in the hospital. **99465** would be used if resuscitation was needed.

4. **D) 99403**

   Explanation: 99403 is used for preventive medicine counseling with a duration of 30 minutes. This service is provided to individuals who, though currently healthy, have risk factors such as family history of disease and seek advice to prevent complications.

5. **A) 99291**

   Explanation: 99291 is used for the first 30-74 minutes of critical care. Since the physician provided 40 minutes of critical care, **99291** is the appropriate code.

6. **B) 99360**

   Explanation: 99360 is used for standby services, where the physician is present but does not actively participate in the care unless needed. The code is time-based, and since the pediatrician was present for more than 30 minutes, **99360** is appropriate.

7. **B) 99204**

   Explanation: 99204 is used for new patients with a moderate level of MDM and 45-59 minutes of total time. Since the physician spent 50 minutes with moderate MDM, **99204** is the correct code.

8. **C) 99211**

   Explanation: 99211 is used for an established patient when the service is provided by clinical staff under the supervision of a physician. This code does not require MDM or time documentation.

9. **A) 99442**

   Explanation: 99441 is used for a 5-10 minute telephone evaluation and management service. Since the physician provided 15 minutes of consultation, **99441** is the correct code. However, if the time was documented as 15-20 minutes, **99442** would be used.

10. **A) 99466, 99467**

    Explanation: 99466 is used for the first 30 minutes of face-to-face critical care during transport, and **99467** is used for each additional 30 minutes. Since the transport took 50 minutes, both **99466** and **99467** are reported.

Chapter 12

Pathology – Coding Guidelines (80000)

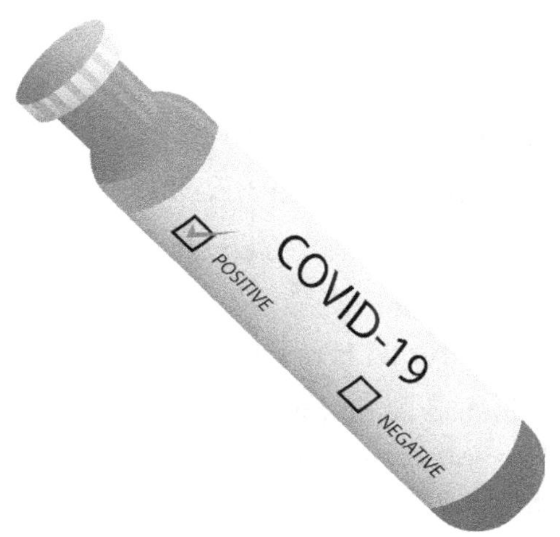

Pathology – Study of diseases

i. Qualitative Test – A test determining the presence or absence of a substance.

ii. Quantitative Test – If a person has a test result indicating a blood alcohol level 0.5

Modifiers only related to pathology and laboratory

i. 90 – Reference or Outside Laboratory. Billed by a physician but performed by an outside Laboratory.

ii. 91 – Repeat clinical diagnostic lab tests. The test should be conducted on the same day and should be repeated because of any kind of error.

iii. 92 – Alternative laboratory platform testing. For example, portable kit (test might be done at home, doctor's office or laboratory). It is single use disposable chamber.

iv. QW – CLIA waived

v. CLIA – Clinical laboratory Improvement Amendment. CMS issues a waiver, if the doctor performs in his office one of the 80 (mentioned) tests because of little risk of error. In such cases use modifier QW.

vi. 99 – Multiple modifier.

Pathology – Coding Guidelines

i. **Do not report E&M codes with pathology chapter codes.**

ii. Do not code surgery chapters codes with pathology codes.

iii. Modifier 51 is not used in pathology codes. Eliminate the option instantly if **modifier 51** is used with pathology codes.

iv. When the doctor is doing repeat test on the same day at different time intervals, use modifier 91 for more than 1 test. However, do not use modifier 91, for tests without physician's order or the repeat test is done because of technician's fault.

v. Modifier 76 is meant for service or procedure code, it is never appended with laboratory codes.

vi. According to CPT coding guidelines, modifier 26 is appended whenever the pathologist is not employed by the facility and is billing separately.

vii. Tests that determines the presence or absence of a drug is referred as Qualitative.

viii. A quantitative test indicates how much analyte is present.

Panel Code – Guidelines

i. When you code a panel like 80047, 80048, 80051 etc. make sure all tests are included in the panel.

ii. Even if a single test is missing you cannot choose the panel and all tests will be coded separately.

iii. Do not use modifier 51 or 52 with panel codes, these are surgery modifiers and cannot be used in laboratory tests.

iv. Panel having the exact same tests cannot be coded twice.

v. If any test is performed separately from panel code then code it separately along with the panel code.

vi. If a group of tests are present in two panel codes, code the panel with the highest number of tests. If there are codes pending then code them separately along with the panel.

QUIZ

1. A lab performs a basic metabolic panel (80048) and later the same day repeats the serum creatinine test (82565) due to an abnormal result. How should this be coded?

   A) 80048
   B) 80048, 82565-91
   C) 80048-91, 82565
   D) 80048, 82565-76

2. A comprehensive metabolic panel (80053) and a lipid panel (80061) are performed on the same day. Which is the correct coding approach?

   A) 80053, 80061
   B) 80053-91, 80061
   C) 80053, 80061-51
   D) 80053, 80061-52

3. A physician orders a hepatic function panel (80076) but requires a repeat bilirubin test (82247) later in the day. How should this be coded?

   A) 80076
   B) 80076, 82247-91
   C) 80076-91, 82247
   D) 80076, 82247-52

4. A patient undergoes a lipid panel (80061) using a portable kit in the physician's office. What is the correct coding?

   A) 80061-90
   B) 80061-91
   C) 80061-92
   D) 80061-QW

5. A renal function panel (80069) is performed, and the BUN test (84520) is repeated due to a technical issue. How should this be coded?

   A) 80069
   B) 80069, 84520-91
   C) 80069, 84520-92
   D) 80069, 84520-76

6. A thyroid panel (80076) and a repeat T4 test (84436) are performed on the same day using a CLIA-waived test kit. What is the correct coding?

   A) 80076, 84436-91
   B) 80076-QW, 84436-91
   C) 80076-92, 84436-92
   D) 80076-QW, 84436-92

7. A general health panel (80050) is performed alongside a renal function panel (80069). Some tests overlap. How should these be coded?

   A) 80050, 80069
   B) 80050, 80069-91
   C) 80050, 80069-52
   D) 80050, additional tests from 80069

8. A physician orders a lipid panel (80061) and then requests an additional CRP test (86140) later in the day. How should this be coded?

   A) 80061
   B) 80061, 86140
   C) 80061-91, 86140
   D) 80061, 86140-52

9. A basic metabolic panel (80048) and a CBC with differential (85025) are performed on the same day. What is the correct coding approach?

    A) 80048, 85025
    B) 80048-91, 85025
    C) 80048, 85025-52
    D) 80048, 85025-51

10. A lipid panel (80061) and an additional triglycerides test (84478) are ordered and performed on the same day. How should this be coded?

    A) 80061
    B) 80061, 84478
    C) 80061-91, 84478
    D) 80061, 84478-52

KEY ANSWERS

1. **B) 80048, 82565-91**

   Explanation: The basic metabolic panel (80048) includes the serum creatinine test (82565). Since the creatinine test is repeated on the same day, the repeat test is coded separately using the 82565 code with modifier 91 to indicate that it was a repeat clinical diagnostic lab test.

2. **A) 80053, 80061**

   Explanation: Both the comprehensive metabolic panel (80053) and the lipid panel (80061) are distinct and do not overlap in tests. Therefore, both panels are coded separately without any modifiers.

3. **B) 80076, 82247-91**

   Explanation: The hepatic function panel (80076) includes the bilirubin test (82247). Since the bilirubin test is repeated later the same day, you should code the repeat test separately using 82247 with modifier 91.

4. **D) 80061-QW**

   Explanation: The use of a portable kit for the lipid panel requires the CLIA waiver, so the appropriate modifier is QW, indicating a CLIA-waived test.

5. **B) 80069, 84520-91**

   Explanation: The renal function panel (80069) includes the BUN test (84520). If the BUN test is repeated on the same day due to a technical issue, it should be coded separately with modifier 91.

6. **B) 80076-QW, 84436-91**

    Explanation: The thyroid panel (80076) is performed using a CLIA-waived test kit, so modifier QW is appended. Since the T4 test (84436) is repeated on the same day, it is coded separately with modifier 91.

7. **D) 80050, additional tests from 80069**

    Explanation: Since there is an overlap in the tests included in 80050 and 80069, the panel with the most tests (80050) should be coded, and any additional tests from 80069 that are not included in 80050 should be coded separately.

8. **B) 80061, 86140**

    Explanation: The lipid panel (80061) and the CRP test (86140) are different tests. They are both coded separately with no need for modifiers since there is no overlap or repeat testing.

9. **A) 80048, 85025**

    Explanation: The basic metabolic panel (80048) and CBC with differential (85025) are distinct panels with no overlap. Both are coded separately without modifiers.

10. **B) 80061, 84478**

    Explanation: The lipid panel (80061) includes the triglycerides test (84478). However, if the triglycerides test is ordered separately, it should be coded in addition to the panel code without any modifiers.

Chapter 13

International Classification of Disease (ICD) – Coding Guidelines

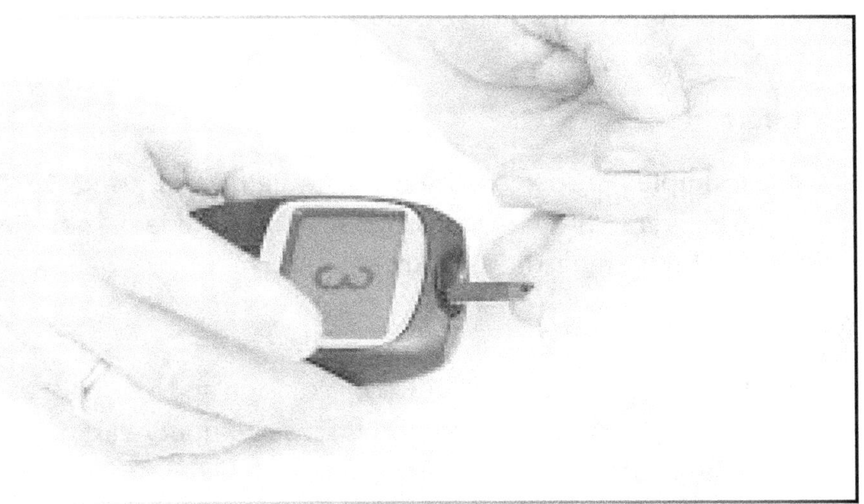

1. **Use the Most Specific Code Available:**

   o **Example:** If a patient has Type 2 Diabetes Mellitus with diabetic neuropathy, use **E11.40** (Type 2 diabetes mellitus with diabetic neuropathy) rather than just **E11.9** (Type 2 diabetes mellitus without complications).

2. **Code to the Highest Level of Certainty:**

   o **Example:** If the provider documents "probable" pneumonia, code the symptom, **R06.02** (Shortness of breath), instead of **J18.9** (Pneumonia, unspecified organism).

3. **Sequence Codes Correctly:**

   o **Example:** For a patient with a primary diagnosis of **I50.9** (Heart failure, unspecified) and secondary diagnosis of **J44.9** (Chronic obstructive pulmonary disease, unspecified), sequence **I50.9** first if heart failure is the primary reason for the visit.

4. **Acute vs. Chronic Conditions:**

   o **Example:** If a patient has both acute bronchitis (**J20.9**) and chronic obstructive bronchitis (**J44.0**), code **J20.9** first, followed by **J44.0**.

5. **Laterality:**

   o **Example:** For osteoarthritis of the right knee, use **M17.11** (Unilateral primary osteoarthritis, right knee), not just **M17.9** (Osteoarthritis of knee, unspecified).

6. **Combination Codes:**

   o **Example:** For a patient with hypertension and heart disease, use **I11.9** (Hypertensive heart disease without heart failure) instead of coding them separately.

7. **Manifestation Codes:**

   o **Example:** For diabetic retinopathy, code **E11.319** (Type 2 diabetes mellitus with unspecified diabetic retinopathy without macular edema) and add the appropriate code for the manifestation.

8. **Avoid Using Codes for Historical Conditions:**

   o **Example:** If a patient had a history of myocardial infarction but is now asymptomatic, use **Z86.74** (Personal history of sudden cardiac arrest) rather than **I21** (Acute myocardial infarction).

9. **Complications of Care:**

   o **Example:** For a post-surgical wound infection, use **T81.4XXA** (Infection following a procedure, initial encounter) as the primary code.

10. **Multiple Conditions:**

   o **Example:** If a patient presents with both hypertension (**I10**) and diabetes (**E11.9**), code both conditions.

Guidelines for Specific Conditions

11. **Fever (R50.9):**

   o **Guideline:** Use **R50.9** (Fever, unspecified) for an unspecified fever. For fever due to an infection, code the infection first, e.g., **B34.9** (Viral infection, unspecified), followed by **R50.9**.

12. **Sepsis (A41.9):**

   o **Guideline:** Code the underlying infection first. If the type of infection is unknown, use **A41.9** (Sepsis, unspecified organism).

13. **AIDS/HIV (B20, Z21):**

   o **Guideline:** Use **B20** (Human immunodeficiency virus [HIV] disease) for patients with symptomatic HIV/AIDS. Use **Z21** (Asymptomatic HIV infection status) for those with asymptomatic HIV. Once a patient has developed an HIV-related illness, always use **B20**.

14. **Kidney Stones (N20.0):**

    o **Guideline:** Use **N20.0** (Calculus of kidney) for kidney stones. If there is associated hydronephrosis, also code **N13.2** (Hydronephrosis with renal and ureteral calculous obstruction).

15. **Urinary Tract Infection (UTI) (N39.0):**

    o **Guideline:** Code **N39.0** (Urinary tract infection, site not specified) for an unspecified UTI. If a specific pathogen is identified, also code the organism, e.g., **B96.20** (Unspecified Escherichia coli [E. coli] as the cause of diseases classified elsewhere).

16. **Hypertension (I10-I15):**

    o **Guideline:** Use **I10** (Essential [primary] hypertension) for uncomplicated hypertension. For hypertension with chronic kidney disease, use **I12.9** (Hypertensive chronic kidney disease with stage 1 through stage 4 chronic kidney disease, or unspecified chronic kidney disease).

17. **Diabetes Mellitus (E08-E13):**

    o **Guideline:** Use the appropriate code for the type of diabetes, e.g., **E11.9** (Type 2 diabetes mellitus without complications). If the patient has complications like diabetic nephropathy, use **E11.21** (Type 2 diabetes mellitus with diabetic nephropathy).

18. **Chronic Kidney Disease (CKD) (N18.1-N18.9):**

    o **Guideline:** Code **N18.5** (Chronic kidney disease, stage 5) for Stage 5 CKD. If CKD is due to hypertension, use a combination code like **I12.9**.

19. **Pneumonia (J18.9):**

   o **Guideline:** Use **J18.9** (Pneumonia, unspecified organism) if the organism is not specified. If caused by a specific organism, like Streptococcus, use **J13** (Pneumonia due to Streptococcus pneumoniae).

20. **Acute Respiratory Failure (J96.0-J96.2):**

   o **Guideline:** Use **J96.00** (Acute respiratory failure, unspecified whether with hypoxia or hypercapnia) for unspecified acute respiratory failure. If the failure is chronic, use **J96.10** (Chronic respiratory failure, unspecified whether with hypoxia or hypercapnia).

21. **Chronic Obstructive Pulmonary Disease (COPD) (J44.9):**

   o **Guideline:** Use **J44.9** (Chronic obstructive pulmonary disease, unspecified) for unspecified COPD. For an acute exacerbation, use **J44.1** (COPD with acute exacerbation).

22. **Asthma (J45.909):**

   o **Guideline:** Use **J45.909** (Unspecified asthma, uncomplicated) for asthma without further specification. If the asthma is in acute exacerbation, use **J45.901** (Unspecified asthma, with [acute] exacerbation).

23. **Congestive Heart Failure (CHF) (I50.9):**

   o **Guideline:** Use **I50.9** (Heart failure, unspecified) for unspecified heart failure. If the heart failure is of a specific type, such as systolic, use **I50.20** (Unspecified systolic [congestive] heart failure).

24. **Myocardial Infarction (MI) (I21-I22):**

     o **Guideline:** Use **I21.3** (ST elevation [STEMI] myocardial infarction of unspecified site) for an acute MI. For a subsequent MI within 28 days, use **I22.9** (Subsequent ST elevation [STEMI] myocardial infarction of unspecified site).

25. **Stroke (Cerebrovascular Accident, CVA) (I63):**

     o **Guideline:** Use **I63.9** (Cerebral infarction, unspecified) for an unspecified ischemic stroke. For sequelae of a stroke, use **I69.3** (Sequelae of cerebral infarction).

26. **Cancer (C00-D49):**

     o **Guideline:** Code the primary malignancy first, e.g., **C34.90** (Malignant neoplasm of unspecified part of unspecified bronchus or lung). For metastasis, add secondary codes, e.g., **C79.51** (Secondary malignant neoplasm of bone).

27. **Anaemia (D64.9):**

     o **Guideline:** Use **D64.9** (Anaemia, unspecified) if the type of anaemia is not specified. For iron deficiency anaemia, use **D50.9** (Iron deficiency anaemia, unspecified).

28. **Fractures (S00-T88):**

     o **Guideline:** Always use a seventh character to indicate the episode of care for fractures. For example, **S52.509A** (Unspecified fracture of the lower end of the right radius, initial encounter for closed fracture).

29. **Gastrointestinal Bleeding (K92.2):**

     o **Guideline:** Use **K92.2** (Gastrointestinal haemorrhage, unspecified) for unspecified GI bleeding. If the bleeding source is known, code it first, e.g., **K25.4** (Chronic or unspecified gastric ulcer with hemorrhage).

30. **Mental Health Conditions (F20-F48):**

o **Guideline:** Code the specific mental health condition first, e.g., **F32.9** (Major depressive disorder, single episode, unspecified). If there are associated symptoms, such as anxiety, code them as well, e.g., **F41.1** (Generalized anxiety disorder).

QUIZ

1. A patient is diagnosed with Type 2 Diabetes Mellitus with diabetic nephropathy. The medical record specifies that the patient also has chronic kidney disease, stage 3. Which codes should be used to accurately capture the patient's condition?

    A) E11.22, N18.3
    B) E11.40, N18.3
    C) E11.21, N18.3
    D) E11.40, N18.9

2. If a patient is diagnosed with an acute myocardial infarction (MI) of the anterior wall and it is noted to be a subsequent MI within 28 days, which code combination should be used?

    A) I21.01, I22.0
    B) I21.09, I22.0
    C) I21.11, I22.1
    D) I21.03, I22.9

3. A patient presents with symptoms of a fever and has been diagnosed with an unspecified viral infection. What is the appropriate coding sequence?

    A) R50.9, B34.9
    B) B34.9, R50.9
    C) R50.9
    D) B34.9

4. A patient is diagnosed with chronic obstructive pulmonary disease (COPD) with an acute exacerbation. Which codes are appropriate?

    A) J44.9, J44.1
    B) J44.1, J44.9
    C) J44.0, J44.1
    D) J44.9

5. For a patient who had a prior history of myocardial infarction but is currently asymptomatic, which code should be used to reflect the past condition?

    A) I21.9
    B) I25.9
    C) I21.4
    D) Z86.74

6. If a patient is diagnosed with chronic kidney disease, stage 2, and hypertension, which codes should be used, and which should be listed first?

    A) I12.0, N18.2
    B) N18.2, I10
    C) I10, N18.2
    D) I12.9, N18.2

7. For a patient with diabetes mellitus type 1 and a history of diabetic retinopathy without macular edema, which code should be used?

    A) E10.359
    B) E11.359
    C) E10.359, E11.359
    D) E10.319

8. A patient is admitted for an acute stroke and is documented to have a cerebral infarction of the right hemisphere. Which code should be used?

    A) I63.9
    B) I63.30
    C) I63.31
    D) I63.40

9. A patient presents with severe iron deficiency anaemia and no other specific symptoms are mentioned. What is the most appropriate code?

   A) D50.0
   B) D50.9
   C) D64.9
   D) D50.8

10. A patient is admitted with an initial encounter for a fracture of the left femur. The fracture is closed and has been diagnosed as a simple fracture. What code should be used?

   A) S72.001A
   B) S72.002A
   C) S72.101A
   D) S72.000A

KEY ANSWERS

1. **C) E11.21, N18.3**

   Solution: Use **E11.21** for Type 2 Diabetes Mellitus with diabetic nephropathy. For chronic kidney disease, stage 3, use **N18.3**. **E11.40** is used for diabetic neuropathy without specifying kidney involvement, and **N18.9** is used for unspecified CKD, which does not accurately reflect the stage.

2. **A) I21.01, I22.0**

   Solution: I21.01 refers to ST elevation (STEMI) of the anterior wall. Since it's a subsequent MI within 28 days, use **I22.0** (Subsequent ST elevation [STEMI] myocardial infarction of anterior wall).

3. **B) B34.9, R50.9**

   Solution: Code the specific condition first, **B34.9** (Viral infection, unspecified), and then code the symptom **R50.9** (Fever, unspecified). This ensures that the viral infection is identified before the symptom.

4. **B) J44.1, J44.9**

   Solution: J44.1 should be used for COPD with acute exacerbation, and **J44.9** should be used if there is additional information or the condition is unspecified. The correct sequence is **J44.1** first, then **J44.9** if needed.

5. **D) Z86.74**

   Solution: Z86.74 (Personal history of sudden cardiac arrest) is used to indicate a past history of myocardial infarction when the patient is asymptomatiC) **I21.9** and **I25.9** reflect current or ongoing conditions.

6. **A) I12.0, N18.2**

    Solution: I12.0 (Hypertension with stage 1 through stage 4 CKD) should be listed first for hypertension with CKD. **N18.2** (Chronic kidney disease, stage 2) should follow if additional specificity is required.

7. **A) E10.359**

    Solution: Use **E10.359** (Type 1 diabetes mellitus with unspecified diabetic retinopathy without macular edema). **E11.359** is for Type 2 diabetes and should not be used in this case.

8. **C) I63.31**

    Solution: I63.31 (Cerebral infarction due to embolism of right middle cerebral artery) accurately describes an acute stroke with a right hemisphere infarction. **I63.30** is for unspecified cerebral infarction, and **I63.40** is for unspecified cerebral infarction without the specific detail.

9. **B) D50.9**

    Solution: **D50.9** (Iron deficiency anemia, unspecified) is appropriate for severe iron deficiency anemia when no other details are provided. **D50.0** is used for iron deficiency anemia due to blood loss, **D64.9** is for anemia unspecified, and **D50.8** is for other specified iron deficiency anemias.

10. **A) S72.001A**

    Solution: S72.001A (Fracture of the left femur, initial encounter for closed fracture) is the correct code for a simple, closed fracture of the left femur with an initial encounter.

Chapter 14

HCPCS – Coding Guidelines

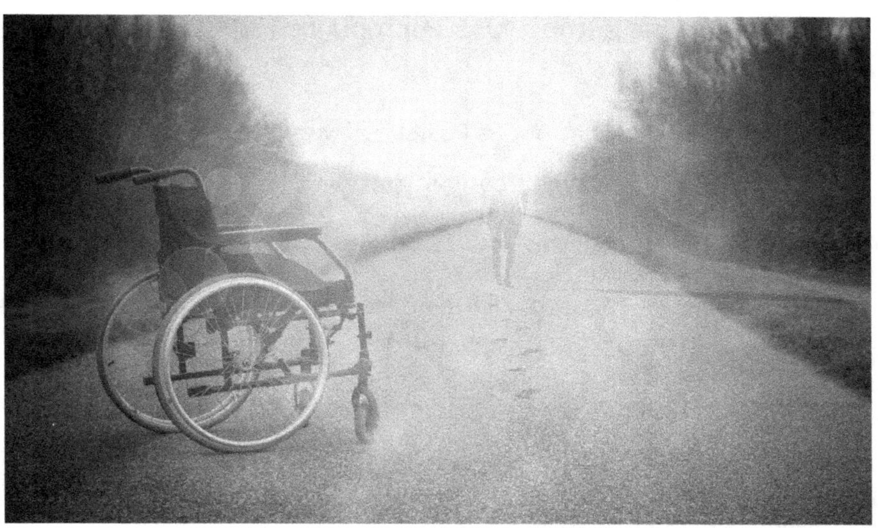

1. HCPCS Level II Code Structure

- **Format**: Alphanumeric codes beginning with a letter followed by four digits (e.g., A1234).

- **Categories**: Includes codes for products, supplies, and services not covered by CPT codes.

2. Modifier Usage

- **Modifiers**: HCPCS Level II codes often require specific modifiers to provide additional detail. For instance:

  - **KX**: Indicates that the requirements specified in the medical policy have been met.

- o **LT/RT**: Denotes left or right side of the body, used with certain codes to specify the location of a service or item.

- o **GA**: Used to indicate that a waiver of liability statement has been issued to the patient.

3. **Durable Medical Equipment (DME)**

- **Coding**: When coding for DME, ensure that the item is necessary for the patient's condition and that it is used in the home setting. Use appropriate HCPCS Level II codes such as:

  - o **E0601**: Continuous Positive Airway Pressure (CPAP) device.

  - o **E1390**: Oxygen concentrator.

4. **Prosthetics and Orthotics**

- **Codes**: HCPCS Level II includes specific codes for prosthetics and orthotics. For example:

  - o **L1950**: Custom-fabricated lower extremity orthosis.

  - o **L8500**: Breast prosthesis, silicone gel or equal.

5. **Drugs and Biologicals**

- **Coding**: Use HCPCS Level II codes for drugs and biologicals administered outside of the physician's office. Examples include:

  - o **J0120**: Injection, methotrexate, 1 mg.

  - o **J2300**: Injection, filgrastim, 300 mcg.

6. **Supplies and Services**

- **Items**: Codes for supplies and services not included in CPT codes. For example:

- o **A4215**: Needles, sterile, hypodermic, any size, each.
- o **S0201**: Home health service provided in the patient's home.

7. **Non-Covered Services**

- **Documentation**: Ensure documentation supports the necessity of services or items. If the service or item is not covered, use appropriate modifiers to indicate patient responsibility. For example:
  - o **GA**: Waiver of liability.
  - o **GZ**: Item or service expected to be denied as not reasonable and necessary.

8. **Bundling and Unbundling**

- **Bundling**: Certain services or supplies may be bundled into one HCPCS code. Avoid unbundling items that are appropriately coded as a single unit.

9. **Proper Coding Practices**

- **Verify**: Always verify the code against the most current HCPCS Level II manual or database.
- **Updates**: HCPCS codes are updated annually. Be aware of changes to ensure accurate coding.
- **Coding Accuracy**: Use the most specific code available to accurately describe the service or item provided.

10. **Claims Submission**

- **Correct Coding**: Ensure that codes are accurate and supported by documentation before submission.

- **Modifiers**: Use modifiers correctly to avoid claim denials or delays.

11. **Correct Use of Modifiers**

    - **Usage**: Apply appropriate modifiers to indicate the specifics of a service or item, such as:

        o **QW**: CLIA waived test.

        o **PD**: Used for physical therapy services provided in a patient's home.

12. **Documentation Requirements**

    - **Support**: Ensure that all claims and codes are supported by proper documentation, including patient records and justifications for DME or other items.

13. **Temporary Codes**

    - **Use**: Be aware of temporary codes (e.g., C codes for outpatient hospital services) and their specific use cases.

14. **Emergency Use Codes**

    - **Specificity**: Use specific codes for emergency items or services provided in urgent situations. For example:

        o **J9999**: Not otherwise classified drug.

15. **Billing for Multiple Items**

    - **Accurate Billing**: When billing for multiple items or services, ensure that each is correctly coded and justified.

16. **Preventing Fraud and Abuse**

    - **Compliance**: Follow all guidelines to prevent fraud and abuse, such as billing for services not provided or misrepresenting services.

17. **Use of HCPCS Codes with CPT Codes**

- **Avoid Mixing**: Do not mix HCPCS Level II codes with CPT codes when coding for a single service or item.

18. **Modifiers for DME**

- **Specific Modifiers**: For DME items, use modifiers like **KX** to indicate compliance with coverage requirements.

19. **International Coding Updates**

- **Understand**: Stay updated with coding changes that might affect international billing or coverage.

20. **Correct Coding Initiative (CCI) Edits**

- **Compliance**: Ensure compliance with CCI edits to avoid incorrect coding and billing.

21. **Use of NDC Codes**

- **National Drug Codes**: Use NDC codes when appropriate for drug identification and billing.

22. **Code Grouping**

- **Combinations**: Use appropriate code combinations for grouped services or items.

23. **Reporting Errors**

- **Reporting**: Report any discovered coding errors promptly to ensure correct billing.

24. **Patient Responsibility Codes**

- **Accuracy**: Accurately code patient responsibility for non-covered services or items.

25. **Educational Materials**

   - **Review**: Continuously review HCPCS educational materials to stay updated on guidelines and changes.

26. **Billing for Supplies**

   - **Appropriate Codes**: Use correct HCPCS codes for medical supplies, including disposables and reusable items.

27. **Patient Diagnosis**

   - **Linking**: Ensure that HCPCS codes are linked correctly to the patient's diagnosis for accurate coding and billing.

28. **Services in Different Settings**

   - **Setting-Specific Codes**: Use different codes for services provided in various settings, such as home vs. hospital.

29. **Regular Audits**

   - **Audits**: Perform regular audits of HCPCS coding practices to ensure accuracy and compliance with current guidelines.

QUIZ

1. A patient requires the use of a continuous positive airway pressure (CPAP) device for sleep apnea. The device is medically necessary and will be used in the patient's home. Which HCPCS code should be used, and what modifier might be necessary if documentation needs to affirm compliance with coverage requirements?

    A) E1390 - No Modifier
    B) E0601 – KX
    C) A4215 – LT
    D) E0601 – LT

2. A physician administers an injection of methotrexate for the treatment of rheumatoid arthritis. Which HCPCS code is appropriate, and which modifier should be used if the injection is administered twice in one day due to a physician's directive?

    A) J0120 – 76
    B) J0120 – 91
    C) J2300 – 76
    D) J0120 – 51

3. When coding for durable medical equipment (DME) that is used in a patient's home, which of the following statements is true?

    A) You should always use modifier LT or RT with DME codes to indicate the side of the body.
    B) DME codes do not require any modifiers when used in a home setting.
    C) The KX modifier is often used with DME codes to indicate that coverage requirements have been met.
    D) DME codes can be billed multiple times on the same day without any modifiers.

4. A patient is provided with a silicone breast prosthesis after a mastectomy. Which HCPCS code should be used, and is there a need for a specific modifier if it is the initial prosthesis?

   A) L8500 – LT
   B) L1950 – RT
   C) L8500 - No Modifier
   D) L8500 – KX

5. Which HCPCS code should be used for a home health service provided in a patient's home, and which modifier would be appropriate if the service is provided on the left side of the body?

   A) S0201 – LT
   B) S0201 – RT
   C) J0120 – LT
   D) S0201 - No Modifier

6. A physician provides a service that is not covered by insurance, and a waiver of liability is issued to the patient. Which modifier should be appended to the HCPCS code to indicate that the patient has accepted financial responsibility?

   A) GA
   B) KX
   C) GZ
   D) QW

KEY ANSWERS

1. **B) E0601 – KX**

   Explanation: The correct HCPCS code for a CPAP device is **E0601**. The **KX** modifier is used to indicate that the requirements specified in the medical policy have been met, confirming that the device is medically necessary and appropriate.

2. **A) J0120 – 76**

   Explanation: The HCPCS code **J0120** corresponds to an injection of methotrexate. The **76** modifier is used to indicate that the procedure (injection) was repeated on the same day due to the physician's directive. The **91** modifier is not appropriate here as it is specific to laboratory tests.

3. **C) The KX modifier is often used with DME codes to indicate that coverage requirements have been met.**

   Explanation: The **KX** modifier is commonly used with DME codes to affirm that the item meets the necessary coverage criteria. **LT/RT** modifiers are used when the equipment is specific to one side of the body but are not mandatory for all DME codes.

4. **C) L8500 - No Modifier**

   Explanation: **L8500** is the correct code for a silicone breast prosthesis. There is no need for a modifier if it is the initial prosthesis being provided. **LT/RT** modifiers are generally used for items that are specific to one side of the body, but in this context, it is unnecessary.

5. **A) S0201 – LT**

    Explanation: S0201 is the correct HCPCS code for home health services provided in a patient's home. If the service is specifically provided on the left side of the body, the **LT** modifier should be used to indicate this.

6. **A) GA**

    Explanation: The **GA** modifier is used when a waiver of liability has been issued to the patient, indicating that the patient understands that the service is not covered by insurance and has accepted financial responsibility. **GZ** is used when no waiver was obtained, and **QW** indicates a CLIA-waived test.

Chapter 15

2026 Revised Medical Coding Guidelines

CPT 2026 — Master Summary

Category	Count	Effective
Total new CPT codes	288	January 1, 2026
Total revised CPT codes	46	January 1, 2026
Total deleted CPT codes	84	January 1, 2026

CPT 2026 — Evaluation & Management (Book Chapter 11)

New Codes Introduced

Code	Description	Status
99445	Supply of device and daily recording/ transmission for remote physiologic monitoring — 2 to 15 days within a 30-day period	Introduced 2026
99470	Remote physiologic monitoring treatment management — first 10 minutes per calendar month	Introduced 2026

Revised Codes

Code	What Changed	Status
99453	Descriptor revised — aligned with new shorter-duration RPM framework	**Revised 2026**
99454	Descriptor revised — now covers supply of device for 16–30 days per month (standard) vs the new shorter-duration code 99445	**Revised 2026**
99457	Descriptor revised as a result of new 99470 being introduced for 10-min treatment management	**Revised 2026**
+99458	Add-on descriptor revised — each additional 20 minutes of RPM treatment management	**Revised 2026**

Note: Core office/outpatient E/M codes 99202–99215, hospital codes 99221–99236, and critical care codes 99291–99292 are all unchanged.

CPT 2026 — Cardiovascular Surgery (Book Chapter 5)

New Codes Introduced

Code	Description	Status
92930	Percutaneous coronary intervention (PCI) — stent placement in 2 or more distinct coronary lesions or bifurcation lesions requiring intervention in both main artery and side branch	**Introduced 2026**
33882	Endovascular repair of thoracic aorta — branched endograft multipiece system with fenestration for left subclavian artery stent graft(s)	**Introduced 2026**
35602	Bypass graft, other than vein — carotid to contralateral carotid (cross-carotid revascularization)	**Introduced 2026**

Code	Description	Status
64654	Baroreflex Activation Therapy (BAT) — implantation of pulse generator	Introduced 2026
64655	BAT — replacement of pulse generator	Introduced 2026
64656	BAT — revision of electrode	Introduced 2026
64657	BAT — removal of electrode	Introduced 2026
64658	BAT — removal of pulse generator	Introduced 2026
64659	BAT — interrogation and programming of pulse generator	Introduced 2026
37254–37299	Lower Extremity Revascularization (LER) — 46 new territory-based codes replacing the deleted legacy codes. Organised by 4 vascular territories: Iliac, Femoral/Popliteal, Tibial/Peroneal, and Inframalleolar. Distinguish straightforward vs complex lesions.	Introduced 2026

Revised Codes

Code	What Changed	Status
33880	Thoracic endovascular aortic repair (TEVAR) — descriptor revised to reflect anatomy-based selection	Revised 2026
33881	TEVAR — descriptor revised	Revised 2026
33883	TEVAR — descriptor revised	Revised 2026
33886	TEVAR — descriptor revised	Revised 2026

Deleted Codes

Code	Description Deleted	Status
33884	TEVAR — deleted, replaced by new code 33882	Deleted 2026
33889	TEVAR — deleted	Deleted 2026
33891	TEVAR — deleted	Deleted 2026
37220	Revascularization, endovascular, iliac artery — deleted; replaced by new LER family 37254–37299	Deleted 2026
37221	Revascularization, iliac artery, with stent — deleted	Deleted 2026
37222	Revascularization, iliac artery, additional vessel — deleted	Deleted 2026
37223	Revascularization, iliac artery, additional vessel with stent — deleted	Deleted 2026
37224	Revascularization, femoral/popliteal — deleted	Deleted 2026
37225	Revascularization, femoral/popliteal with atherectomy — deleted	Deleted 2026
37226	Revascularization, femoral/popliteal with stent — deleted	Deleted 2026
37227	Revascularization, femoral/popliteal with stent and atherectomy — deleted	Deleted 2026
37228	Revascularization, tibial/peroneal — deleted	Deleted 2026
37229	Revascularization, tibial/peroneal with atherectomy — deleted	Deleted 2026
37230	Revascularization, tibial/peroneal with stent — deleted	Deleted 2026
37231	Revascularization, tibial/peroneal with stent and atherectomy — deleted	Deleted 2026

Code	Description Deleted	Status
37232	Revascularization, tibial/peroneal, each additional — deleted	Deleted 2026
37233	Revascularization, tibial/peroneal, additional with atherectomy — deleted	Deleted 2026
37234	Revascularization, tibial/peroneal, additional with stent — deleted	Deleted 2026
37235	Revascularization, tibial/peroneal, additional with stent and atherectomy — deleted	Deleted 2026

CPT 2026 — Radiology (Book Chapter 9)

New Codes Introduced

Code	Description	Status
70471	CT Angiography (CTA) of the head and neck with contrast; bundles images without contrast and all image postprocessing in the same session	Introduced 2026
+70472	CT cerebral perfusion — add-on code when performed in same session as head CT or head/neck CTA of same anatomy	Introduced 2026
70473	CT cerebral perfusion — standalone code when performed without a concurrent head CT or head/neck CTA	Introduced 2026
0877T	CT-based AI diagnostic classification — interstitial lung disease (Category III)	Introduced 2026
0878T	CT-based AI diagnostic classification — interstitial lung disease, add-on (Category III)	Introduced 2026
0879T	CT-based AI diagnostic classification — interstitial lung disease, additional (Category III)	Introduced 2026

Code	Description	Status
0880T	CT-based AI diagnostic classification — interstitial lung disease, additional (Category III)	**Introduced 2026**
0898T	Noninvasive prostate estimation mapping using AI analysis (Category III)	**Introduced 2026**
0992T	Analysis of perivascular fat to assess cardiac risk (Category III)	**Introduced 2026**
0993T	Analysis of perivascular fat with concurrent CT scan to assess cardiac risk (Category III)	**Introduced 2026**
0710T	Coronary atherosclerosis quantification analysis — noninvasive arterial plaque analysis (Category I)	**Introduced 2026**

Revised Codes

Code	What Changed	Status
77402	Radiation treatment delivery — revised to represent Level 1 (simple); image guidance and motion management now bundled into delivery codes	**Revised 2026**
77407	Radiation treatment delivery — revised to represent Level 2 (intermediate)	**Revised 2026**
77412	Radiation treatment delivery — revised to represent Level 3 (complex)	**Revised 2026**

Note: Radiation treatment management code 77427 (per 5 fractions) is unchanged.

CPT 2026 — Pathology & Laboratory (Book Chapter 12)

New Codes Introduced

Code	Description	Status
82233	Beta-amyloid 1-40 (Abeta 40) — biomarker for Alzheimer's disease	Introduced 2026
82234	Beta-amyloid 1-42 (Abeta 42) — biomarker for Alzheimer's disease	Introduced 2026
83884	Neurofilament light chain (NfL) — tracks disease progression in multiple sclerosis and neurodegenerative conditions	Introduced 2026
84393	Tau, phosphorylated (e.g., pTau 181, pTau 217) — each; biomarker for Alzheimer's	Introduced 2026
84395	Tau — additional specificity variant for dementia biomarker evaluation	Introduced 2026
86581	Streptococcus pneumoniae antibody (IgG), serotypes, multiplex immunoassay, quantitative	Introduced 2026
87513	Helicobacter pylori (H. pylori), clarithromycin resistance, amplified probe technique	Introduced 2026
87564	Mycobacterium tuberculosis, rifampin resistance, amplified probe technique	Introduced 2026
87594	Pneumocystis jirovecii, amplified probe technique (BAL specimen)	Introduced 2026
87626	Human Papillomavirus (HPV) — separately reported high-risk types (e.g., 16, 18, 31, 45, 51, 52)	Introduced 2026

Note: Panel code rules, Modifier 51 prohibition, and qualitative/ quantitative distinction are all unchanged.

CPT 2026 — Integumentary System (Book Chapter 3)

Revised Code

Code	What Changed	Status
10040	Descriptor revised — 'Acne surgery' replaced with 'Extraction'	**Revised 2026**

CPT 2026 — Musculoskeletal System (Book Chapter 4)

Revised Codes

Code	What Changed	Status
27278	Arthrodesis — editorial revision to code descriptor	**Revised 2026**
27279	Arthrodesis — editorial revision to code descriptor	**Revised 2026**

CPT 2026 — Nervous System (Book Chapter 8)

New Codes Introduced

Code	Description	Status
62330	Percutaneous lumbar decompression via partial removal of ligamentum flavum with image guidance	**Introduced 2026**
62331	Percutaneous lumbar decompression — bilateral	**Introduced 2026**
+63032	Add-on — annular defect repair using bone-anchored closure device with lumbar decompression	**Introduced 2026**
64567	Non-implantable percutaneous electrical nerve field stimulation (PENFS) of cranial nerves	**Introduced 2026**

Code	Description	Status
64728	Percutaneous balloon decompression of the median nerve in carpal tunnel syndrome, including ultrasound guidance	**Introduced 2026**

CPT 2026 — Digestive System (Book Chapter 6)

New Code Introduced

Code	Description	Status
43889	Endoscopic Sleeve Gastroplasty (ESG) — transoral endoscopic suturing to reduce stomach volume	**Introduced 2026**

ICD-10-CM FY2026 — All Key Code Changes

Effective October 1, 2025. Total changes: **487 new**, **38 revised**, **28 deleted** diagnosis codes.

ICD-10-CM 2026 — New Injury Codes (Book Chapter 13, S-Codes)

Over 213 of the new ICD-10-CM codes are in Chapter 19 (Injury, S00–T88), adding anatomical specificity and laterality. The following are the key new codes directly referenced in Chapter 15 of the book:

New Code	Description	Status
S30.11	Contusion of abdominal wall	**Added FY2026**
S30.12	Contusion of groin	**Added FY2026**
S30.13	Contusion of flank	**Added FY2026**
R10.2-	Pelvic and perineal pain — converted to parent code with 16 new sub-codes for specificity in pain/tenderness of pelvic, perineal, subpubic, abdominal, and flank areas	**Added FY2026**

New Code	Description	Status
R11.16	Cannabis hyperemesis syndrome (CHS)	**Added FY2026**

ICD-10-CM 2026 — Key New Diagnosis Codes by System

New Code	Description	Status
E11.A	Type 2 diabetes mellitus without complications in remission — requires provider to document exact term 'remission'	**Added FY2026**
G35.A-	Multiple sclerosis — relapsing-remitting type (replaces deleted G35)	**Added FY2026**
G35.B-	Multiple sclerosis — primary progressive type (replaces deleted G35)	**Added FY2026**
G35.C-	Multiple sclerosis — secondary progressive type (replaces deleted G35)	**Added FY2026**
N00.B1	Acute nephritic syndrome with idiopathic immune complex membranoproliferative glomerulonephritis (IC-MPGN)	**Added FY2026**
N00.B2	Acute nephritic syndrome with secondary IC-MPGN	**Added FY2026**
N04.B1	Nephrotic syndrome with idiopathic IC-MPGN	**Added FY2026**
N04.B2	Nephrotic syndrome with secondary IC-MPGN	**Added FY2026**
N07.B	Hereditary nephropathy — APOL1-mediated kidney disease (AMKD)	**Added FY2026**
M05.A	Abnormal rheumatoid factor and anti-citrullinated protein antibody with rheumatoid arthritis	**Added FY2026**

New Code	Description	Status
C50.A-	Malignant inflammatory neoplasm of breast (IBC) — three new sub-codes for inflammatory breast cancer	**Added FY2026**
W44.A9	Other batteries entering into or through a natural orifice	**Added FY2026**
Z40.81	Encounter for prophylactic surgery for removal of ovary(s) — persons without known genetic/familial risk factors	**Added FY2026**
Z40.82	Encounter for prophylactic surgery for removal of fallopian tube(s) — persons without known genetic/familial risk factors	**Added FY2026**
L98.435	Non-pressure chronic ulcer of abdomen with muscle involvement without evidence of necrosis	**Added FY2026**
L98.436	Non-pressure chronic ulcer of abdomen with bone involvement without evidence of necrosis	**Added FY2026**
L98.438	Non-pressure chronic ulcer of abdomen with other specified severity	**Added FY2026**

ICD-10-CM 2026 — Deleted Codes

Deleted Code	Description	Replaced By
G35	Multiple sclerosis — general/ unspecified code deleted	**Replaced by G35.A-, G35.B-, G35.C- (specific MS phenotype required)**
N00.5	Acute nephritic syndrome with membranoproliferative glomerulonephritis types 1 and 3 or NOS	**Replaced by N00.B1 and N00.B2**

Deleted Code	Description	Replaced By
N04.5	Nephrotic syndrome with diffuse mesangiocapillary glomerulonephritis — deleted	**Replaced by N04.B1 and N04.B2**
Z40.02	Encounter for prophylactic removal of ovary(s) and fallopian tube(s) — combined code deleted	**Replaced by Z40.81 and Z40.82 (separate codes)**

ICD-10-CM 2026 — Revised Codes

Revised Code	What Changed	Status
J44	COPD — Excludes1 note changed to Excludes2 for emphysema due to inhalation of chemicals/gases/fumes/vapors (J68.4)	**Guideline revised FY2026**
M21.159	Varus deformity, not elsewhere classified — descriptor revised to specify 'unspecified hip'	**Revised FY2026**
M61.129	Myositis ossificans progressiva — descriptor revised to clarify applies to right or left upper arm	**Revised FY2026**
Z01	Encounter for other special examination — Excludes1 changed to Excludes2 for pregnancy/reproduction examinations	**Revised FY2026**
Z59.86-	Financial insecurity — converted to parent code with 3 new specific sub-codes	**Revised FY2026**

Revised Code	What Changed	Status
Z91.011-	Allergy to milk products — converted to parent with 3 new sub-codes	**Revised FY2026**
Z91.012	Allergy to eggs — converted to parent with 3 new sub-codes	**Revised FY2026**

Note: ICD-10-CM sequencing rules, laterality, 7th character (A/D/S), and combination code rules are all unchanged for FY2026.

HCPCS Level II 2026 — All Key Code Changes

Effective January 1, 2026. Total changes: **160 new codes, 101 deleted codes, ~300 revised descriptors**.

HCPCS 2026 — New A-Codes (Medical Supplies)

New Code	Description	Status
A4295	Intermittent urinary catheter, straight tip, with hydrophilic coating	**Added 2026**
A4296	Intermittent urinary catheter, coude (curved) tip, with hydrophilic coating	**Added 2026**
A4297	Intermittent urinary catheter — third new hydrophilic catheter specification code	**Added 2026**

HCPCS 2026 — New C-Codes (Outpatient Hospital / DME)

New Code	Description	Status
C1607	Implantable integrated neurostimulator	Added 2026
C-codes	19 total new C-codes for various procedures and durable medical equipment	19 codes added 2026

HCPCS 2026 — New G-Codes (Procedures/Services)

New Code	Description	Status
G0568	Psychiatric Collaborative Care Management — initial contact	Added 2026
G0569	Psychiatric Collaborative Care Management — per calendar month	Added 2026
G0570	Psychiatric Collaborative Care Management — additional	Added 2026
G0660– G0668	TEAM remote E/M services — align with CPT E/M codes 99201–99205, 99212–99215	9 codes added 2026
G9871	Online diabetes management service	Added 2026
G2076	Social determinants of health code — descriptor updated; 'Social Determinants of Health' replaced with 'upstream drivers'	Revised 2026
G2077	Same descriptor update — 'Social Determinants of Health' → 'upstream drivers'	Revised 2026

HCPCS 2026 — New J-Codes (Drug Injections)

Several J-codes were introduced for newly FDA-approved drugs. Key examples:

New Code	Description	Status
J9256	Injection, nipocalimab-aahu, 3 mg (crosswalked from deleted C9305)	**Replaces C9305, 2026**
J9326	Injection, telisotuzumab vedotin-tllv, 1 mg (crosswalked from deleted C9306)	**Replaces C9306, 2026**

HCPCS 2026 — New M-Codes (Quality / MIPS Value Pathways)

New Code	Description	Status
M1426–M1503	78 new M-codes for MIPS Value Pathway (MVP) tracking across specialties (e.g., telehealth encounter identification, prostate bone scan documentation, Hepatitis C treatment outcomes, falls risk management)	**78 codes added 2026**
M1427	Documentation of medical reason for performing a bone scan (prostate cancer pain, salvage therapy, or other)	**Added 2026**
M1482–M1485	Hepatitis C — tracking sustained virological response	**Added 2026**
M1492–M1497	Falls Risk Management — differentiates reported fall from documented plan of care	**Added 2026**
M1426, M1431, M1436+	Telehealth encounter identification across different clinical scenarios	**Added 2026**

HCPCS 2026 — New Q-Codes (Biosimilars / Skin Substitutes)

New Code	Description	Status
Q5160	Bevacizumab-nwgd — brand-name biosimilar	**Added 2026**
Q4411	AmnioMatrixF4X — human cell/tissue product, cover and barrier for acute and chronic wounds	**Added 2026**
Q-codes	25 total new Q-codes for biosimilars and skin-substitute products added in 2026	**25 codes added 2026**

HCPCS 2026 — Deleted Codes

Deleted Code	Description	Status
C9305	Injection, nipocalimab-aahu, 3 mg — discontinued temporary C-code	**Replaced by J9256**
C9306	Injection, telisotuzumab vedotin-tllv, 1 mg — discontinued temporary C-code	**Replaced by J9326**
J-codes (multiple)	Numerous J-codes for discontinued, inactive, or no-longer-payable drugs removed to prevent outdated billing	**101 total deletions across J, S, and other codes**
S-codes (select)	Select S-codes crosswalked to newly created J-codes; now billed under Medicare-recognised drug codes	**Included in 101 total deletions**

Note: Modifier rules KX, GA, GZ, QW, LT, RT, JA, JB are all unchanged for 2026. Modifier JA (IV infusion) and JB (subcutaneous injection) continue to be required for J-codes that do not specify route of administration.

SOURCES:

The guidelines and questions are derived from the CPT, ICD, and HCPCS study manuals published by AAPC. These respected sources are cited throughout the chapters to acknowledge their contributions. The content from these manuals has been organized and listed pointwise for the reader's convenience, ensuring that credit is given where it is due. This compilation is created with regard to the original materials, aiming to provide a cohesive and comprehensive reference.

www.ingramcontent.com/pod-product-compliance
Lightning Source LLC
Chambersburg PA
CBHW070832160726
48004CB00001B/348